MORE THAN MEDICINE

A volume in the series
The Culture and Politics of Health Care Work
Edited by Suzanne Gordon and Sioban Nelson

For a list of books in the series, visit our website at
cornellpress.cornell.edu.

MORE THAN MEDICINE

Nurse Practitioners and the Problems
They Solve for Patients, Health Care
Organizations, and the State

LaTonya J. Trotter

ILR PRESS
AN IMPRINT OF CORNELL UNIVERSITY PRESS   ITHACA AND LONDON

First published 2020 by Cornell University Press

Library of Congress Cataloging-in-Publication Data

Names: Trotter, LaTonya J., author.
Title: More than medicine : nurse practitioners and the problems they solve for
    patients, health care organizations, and the state / LaTonya J. Trotter.
Description: Ithaca : ILR Press, an imprint of Cornell University Press, 2020. |
    Series: The culture and politics of health care work | Includes bibliographical
    references and index.
Identifiers: LCCN 2019026554 (print) | LCCN 2019026555 (ebook) |
    ISBN 9781501748141 (hardcover) | ISBN 9781501748158 (paperback) |
    ISBN 9781501748165 (epub) | ISBN 9781501748172 (pdf)
Subjects: LCSH: Nurse practitioners—United States. | Geriatric nursing—
    Social aspects—United States. | Senior centers—United States. |
    Older African Americans—Care. | Older African Americans—Services for.
Classification: LCC RT82.8 .T76 2020 (print) | LCC RT82.8 (ebook) |
    DDC 610.7306/920973—dc23
LC record available at https://lccn.loc.gov/2019026554
LC ebook record available at https://lccn.loc.gov/2019026555

In memoriam
Fannie Weatherspoon Rutley, Ossie Whitfield Trotter, and
Octavia E. Butler

Contents

Acknowledgments

Writing this book was lonely work, but I did not do it alone. From reading drafts to asking questions or sometimes just sharing a well-placed word, a network of people stands behind its production. The support and mentorship I received from Princeton's sociology department were key to the development of this book. The weight of that mentorship fell on the shoulders of Elizabeth M. Armstrong. In addition to her insight, Betsy gave me the gift of freedom. She always supported me in finding my own way. Even as I charged ahead, she was right there with me, moving several small mountains on my behalf. I also thank Mitchell Duneier. Everything I know about fieldwork I learned from him. Without his willingness to share what he knew, I would not have had the confidence to undertake this work.

I am grateful to Katherine Newman. Early in my training, she challenged me, very pointedly, "to not do trivial work." Although she moved on from Princeton before she could see the direction I ultimately took, her words hit their mark and altered my path in the most radical way possible. I also want to express my deep appreciation to Paul DiMaggio, King-To Yeung, and Viviana A. Zelizer at Princeton for their careful reading and incisive questions. Money, of course, matters too. My research was made possible through the support of a Princeton University Graduate Fellowship, a National Science Foundation Graduate Research Fellowship, a National Institutes of Health Demography Traineeship, a Princeton University Woodrow Wilson Scholars Fellowship, and a Princeton University Center for Health and Wellbeing Research Grant.

Princeton gave me solid training as a sociologist, but I had a good deal to learn about being a writer. Anne Vittoria carefully read my first draft, suggesting what could be expanded and what needed to be laid to rest. As I waded into the thick of writing and rewriting, I received feedback leavened with encouragement from many people. Early readers included Pallavi Banerjee, Marzia Milazzo, Michelle Murray, and Jennifer Reich. For their advice, support, and persistent reminders on how to be a sociologist, I thank Amy Kate Bailey, Emily Marshall, Christine Percheski, and Hana Shepherd. Clare Stacey, care work scholar extraordinaire, provided a set of comments that helped me sharpen my arguments and smooth out the rough edges. I also wish to thank The Porch Writers' Collective, a nonprofit writing center in Nashville. I was sustained by its community of writers as well as its workshops. A special word of thanks to Susannah Felts, cofounder of The Porch, for helping me breathe a little life back into my prose. Finally, I am grateful to Dan Cornfield. Thank you for being a good colleague and an even better friend.

Some of the quoted material and argument of chapter 2 appeared in early form in my 2015 work "The Caring Professional? Nurse Practitioners, Social Work, and the Performance of Expertise," within the Rutgers University Press published volume *Caring on the Clock: The Complexities and Contradictions of Paid Care Work*, edited by Mignon Duffy, Amy Armenia, and Clare L. Stacey. Additionally, some of the quotations I include in this book from NPs, physicians, and nursing students first appeared in print, if put to somewhat different use, in my 2019 article "'I'm Not a Doctor. I'm a Nurse': Reparative Boundary-Work in Nurse Practitioner Education," *Social Currents* 6 (2): 105–20, and in my 2017 article "Making A Career: Reproducing Gender within a Predominately Female Profession," *Gender & Society* 31 (4): 503–25.

The editors at Cornell University Press deserve their own mention. I always imagined that writers write and publishers publish. I never knew just how important the folks at a press could be in the writing. Sioban Nelson, one of the editors of this series, gave me important and useful feedback on multiple drafts; more than that, though, she offered encouragement. Even as I took much (much) longer to finish than I predicted, Sioban stood by the work, and in standing by the work she stood by me. I also want to thank Fran Benson, the editorial director at ILR Press, for seeing the glimmer of possibility in my book and sending me over to the series where it found its home.

Finally, I would like to convey my deepest gratitude to all the people who let me spend time with them as I undertook this work. Although they appear in these pages by pseudonyms, I would like each one to know that every hour, every story, every answer given was not wasted. I watched. I listened. And I tried to get it right. I hope they find some version of their own truth within these pages. A special word of thanks is reserved for the members at Forest Grove Elder Services—those who invited me into their homes as well as those who just let me serve them lunch. They opened my eyes to a world I needed to understand. And when I struggled, I drew strength from the ability of these women and men to press on, in spite of a world of obstacles. That feeling of connection, and the responsibility that came with it, was sometimes all that stood between me and giving up. To the people of the Grove, both living and dead, I owe a debt I can never repay.

A Word about Methods

Over the years this book has unfolded, I have often been asked, "How did you become interested in nurse practitioners?" I thought it a strange question. Why is anyone interested in anything? But I soon began to hear the less polite question underneath the one being asked: Why would anyone be interested in nursing? As a society, we profess a deep respect for nursing, but that respect does not usually translate into recognition. If there is a hierarchy of interestingness in health care, physicians are at the top. Nurses are much further down. From *Ben Casey* in the 1960s to *Grey's Anatomy* in the 2000s, we have a seemingly infinite fascination with the work that physicians do. Nurses appear as supportive players, but we see very little of nursing work, which encourages the assumption is that there is little worth seeing.

Sociologists, perhaps, have inadvertently taken their cues from this cultural trend. In 2006, I began my doctoral work in sociology at Princeton University. I had just completed my master's in public health and had embarked on a study of health care from the sociological perspective. As I made my way through the literature on physician education and the roles pharmaceutical companies, malpractice lawyers, and insurance companies increasingly play in shaping the patient encounter, I noticed that something seemed to be missing: nurses. To be fair, they were not wholly absent from sociological accounts (see Anspach 1997; Chambliss 1996; Freidson 1970; Freidson 1988a). However, when scholars wrote about nursing, they were telling the story of nurses. When scholars wrote about physicians, they were telling the story of health care.

This cordoning off of nursing seemed curiously out of sync with reality. By any measure, nurses are not marginal to health care. Without the labor of literally millions of nurses, the work of modern health care would grind to a halt. I was poised to notice this absence through a more personal connection as well. A year before I began my studies at Princeton, my friend Darlene matriculated at Yale School of Nursing. I did not know it at the time, but Yale would become my first, if informal, field site and Darlene, my chief informant. At the age of thirty-seven, Darlene was entering nursing as a second career. She had never considered becoming a bedside nurse; she wanted to become a nurse practitioner (NP). In both our minds, these were two different occupations. Nursing was nursing; becoming an NP was closer to being a physician. There was, however, a practical wrinkle in our view of things. Prospective NPs have to complete the training and licensing process to become a registered nurse (RN). In other words, becoming an NP required learning to be an RN first.

During regular telephone calls, I listened to Darlene struggle through her first year, vacillating between frustration and surprise that these "bedside nursing skills" were not just a credentialing hurdle but a necessary part of how one became a skilled NP. Until that first year, I don't think either of us really understood that NPs were nurses. Darlene found herself not only learning bedside nursing skills but also becoming a nurse in ways neither of us anticipated. As she began talking to me about "the nursing perspective" and explaining how it differed from a physician's approach to patient care, I decided to transition from listening friend to ethnographic observer.

Yale School of Nursing

Every other week, I took the train from Princeton to New Haven to sit in on Darlene's Friday classes. In the evenings, I would study with small groups of students or just sit and talk with Darlene in her studio apartment. It was through these weekend trips that I became aware, as if for the first time, that Darlene was learning diagnostic medicine from nurses. That the faculty who delivered her curriculum were nurses. And that the people who evaluated her mastery of clinical skills were nurses. Through that awareness, I realized my unspoken assumption that the work of NPs was supervised by physicians. But here, in the place where future NPs were being trained, physicians were colleagues and sometimes trusted mentors, but they were certainly not supervisors.

My experience at Yale was formative. Although there were many things I had read about NPs, I did not really come to know the NP until I began to immerse myself in the world of the nursing school. No pseudonym is needed when I speak of my time at Yale. This was not research in the administrative sense of the word. While I asked permission to attend classes, I secured no paper trail of approval to conduct research. Although I spoke with students about their experiences, there were no formal interviews or signed consent forms. And while I took field notes, none of that data appears in the account that follows. Yet I mention it here because it formed the groundwork for this project and was as useful to my understanding of the NP as the descriptions that appear in my published work. Because of the generosity of Darlene, who hosted me, her classmates who spoke with me, and the Yale School of Nursing faculty who opened their classrooms to me, I arrived at an entirely different set of questions to ask about the NP. Instead of beginning with who policy makers thought NPs were or what nursing advocates argued they should be, I began with two core questions: Who did NPs believe themselves to be? And how did they come to that understanding?

Stanton School of Nursing

The time I spent at Yale was integral to forming a set of questions, but it was not enough to answer them. I began a more systematic set of investigations at a different institution: Stanton School of Nursing (a pseudonym). In January of 2009, I began sitting in on classes and university events alongside a fifteen-person cohort of NP students. My observational data included classroom lectures as well as day-to-day conversations with students, faculty, guest lecturers, and Stanton administrators. My classroom observations spanned the last twelve months of a twenty-four-month program. The timing of my observations was strategic; the first twelve months of the curriculum were entirely didactic. It was in the second half that students began trying out their classroom knowledge within clinical placements.

For NP students, the classroom plays a particularly formative role. Nurse practitioner training differs from physician training in many ways, but chief among them is that clinical practice is not completed within residencies where students learn in groups on the wards of a single hospital. Instead, NP students are typically dispersed as individuals to a variety of sites that match their specialties. Those planning to enter family practice, for example, might spend a clinical placement at an urgent care clinic or neighborhood health center. While these placements are the primary sites for clinical skill building, the classroom remains the primary location for collective sense-making. At Stanton, students and faculty would bring stories "back from the field" about patient encounters, information from site preceptors (who might be NPs or MDs), and the practical quandaries of practicing as an NP. The classroom became the place where disparate and contradictory information was reshaped into cohesive narratives of who NPs were, what NPs did, and what NPs knew. In total, I spent 210 hours in direct observation at the nursing school. I also completed formal interviews with ten members of the student cohort.

I left Stanton with a solid understanding of the professional resources that NPs marshaled to understand themselves. However, if I wanted to understand what NPs do, I had to find a site of NP practice. As is often true in fieldwork, serendipity as much as choice led me to Forest Grove Elder Services (a pseudonym). Which is to say, it was not the kind of place I would have chosen. As will soon become clear, little about the Grove is representative of US health care. But

I eventually came to understand, as generations of fieldworkers before me, the value of the aberrant case.

Forest Grove Elder Services

Forest Grove Elder Services is a comprehensive care organization that provides a wide range of medical and supportive services for older adults. It operates as part of a federal demonstration project to assess more cost-effective alternatives to nursing home care. All the Grove's members are at least fifty-five years old and certified as eligible for nursing home care because of a combination of medical frailty, cognitive deficits, and physical impairments. The backbone of the Grove's model of service delivery is a centralized, medically supervised adult day center. Members attend the center one to five days a week in order to receive personal care, primary health care services, social work services, physical and occupational therapy, supervision if they have significant cognitive impairments, and socialization through recreational activities. For my purposes, however, the chief attraction of the Grove was that the majority of its health care was provided by NPs. The Grove identifies as a nurse-managed health care organization; the work of its NPs is a celebrated feature of its organizational structure.

In October of 2009, I began volunteering at the Grove's day center, spending time with members in recreational activities. I would begin and end my days with the members, arriving at the center at ten in the morning and leaving at three thirty or four in the afternoon. I did so two to three days a week for a full year, beginning with a standard schedule of Tuesdays and Thursdays, and eventually sampling additional days for comparison. As a volunteer, I developed a view of the Grove from the members' perspective, as well as an understanding of how staff outside the clinic navigated center life, such as the nurses' aides, the recreational services staff, outside vendors hired by the Grove to provide entertainment, and other volunteers.

In October of 2010, I began seventeen consecutive months of fieldwork focused primarily on the health care that happened at the Grove. Five days a week, I would arrive early enough for the eight forty-five morning meeting and leave with the members in the afternoon. I spent most of this time following the range of providers who gave direct medical care. The NP was the primary provider at the Grove; however, integral to the Grove's model of care was its reliance on interdisciplinary teams. The NPs worked within teams that included physicians, RNs, social workers, physical therapists, and occupational therapists.

I initially concentrated my observations and interviews among the NPs, the RNs, and the physicians because their work was located inside the clinic. After gaining a view of how clinic work was negotiated, I extended my observations and interviews to include the social workers and, to some extent, the occupational therapists, physical therapists, and marketing staff.

In addition to observing individuals, I observed the teams at work through weekly team meetings and the email exchanges that were sent to team lists. During these moments of group decision-making, I had a view of a wider range of actors, including the home care staff, transportation department workers, interns, and fellows. To understand the broader organization of work, I routinely attended other organizational meetings such as daily morning meetings, twice-weekly assessment meetings, and weekly primary care meetings. I attended other meetings less routinely, such as the nurses' meeting, the social work department's meeting, the managers' meeting, and the meeting of the ethics committee.

I tried to spend equal amounts of time with each team, but I minimized observing clinician-patient contact for one. This team drew its patient panel from "atypical" members: those who received only home-based care because of an inability (or sometimes unwillingness) to attend the center, and those who spent their in-center time in the secured Alzheimer's wing on the first floor. My decision was partly for practical reasons—I had my hands full following the teams located in the second floor clinic without following those in the secured wing or those whose care was exclusively home based. But there were also ethical considerations. After sitting in on a few clinical visits with patients with significant cognitive impairments, I felt uncertain of their ability to assent to my presence. I did not, however, entirely exclude this team from my observations; I attended its weekly team meetings and interviewed its clinicians.

Audio recordings have become almost de rigueur for contemporary ethnographers. In a medical setting with health information flowing through the air like mist, this was not an option open to me. Instead, I recorded my observations through written field notes. To some extent, having to handwrite notes is a barrier to recording the exact order and articulation of social life. However, the repeated taking of field notes does allow one to capture the pattern of both physical and verbal behavior. Additionally, there may be something useful about written field notes as an ethical choice in terms of consent. After two and a half years at the Grove, I had become a fixture. It would have been easy to forget my primary role as a researcher and what my presence signaled consent to. The ubiquitous presence of my notebook and the visible activity of my writing was a subtle but ever-present signal that whatever else I might be, I was a researcher.

I did not hide in bathrooms to record surreptitious jottings. With a notebook and ballpoint pen, I wrote notes out in the open.

I have also taken my ethical commitments to consent seriously in other ways. While the Grove gave me access to the work, each person gave me permission to observe their work, for every day I observed, and for every activity I observed. This also meant that some workers did not consent. One of the social workers allowed me to spend one week shadowing her but quickly tired of my presence in her office. Other workers would ask me to leave their offices when they made personal phone calls, had lunch, or just wanted some time away from my silent stares. Others still would consent to my writing information down but ask me not to attribute certain statements to their position in the organization; they knew that the use of a pseudonym would not make them anonymous to their colleagues. But sometimes, my sense of responsibility was to the work itself.

I did not shy away from using unflattering words about colleagues that were said during recorded interviews. A researcher's responsibility to protect subjects does not extend to the right to censor the words that they choose to put on the record. Nor did I censor myself in recording tense exchanges that happened in organizationally public spaces. I went to the Grove to understand intraprofessional conflict and negotiation; when I witnessed it, I wrote it down. Access to the collective work at the Grove was a gift; to not do what I came to do would have been to squander it. Not everyone will agree with the decisions I have made. However, there are too few conversations about the everyday ethics of fieldwork because the decisions made are often hidden from view. In making my decisions transparent, I hope to be a part of future conversations.

The above is an accurate portrayal of the data I collected at the Grove. But I want to take a moment to account for information that is often rendered invisible when one tries to separate "data" from other kinds of evidence. In preparation for my fieldwork, I had read several histories of nursing. Yet I did not fully understand the professional and political meaning of naming nursing work until I began attending nursing and NP conferences. I did not really understand what was meant by "nurse-managed clinic" until I had spent a few days observing and learning how a variety of such places operate.

Even at the Grove, I spent time in locations and with people that do not make much of an appearance in this account. There were the hours I spent with members inside the Grove, through the telephone, and at their homes. These observations and conversations helped me to more fully understand the challenges that the Grove's members faced, not just as patients, but as older adults grappling with racism, poverty, and disability. Without that context, I doubt I would have developed an analysis that placed the NP against the larger backdrop of welfare state retrenchment. There were the hours I spent shadowing the occupational

therapists, physical therapists, bedside nurses, marketing staff, recreational services staff, volunteers, and the chaplain. Although most of these observations are
not documented here, the collective comparisons that they enabled were critical
in helping me distinguish an expansive notion of NP expertise from the expansive version of work that everyone performed as part of the Grove's organizational mission.

MORE THAN MEDICINE

Introduction

At the beginning of each day, over one hundred older adults arrive at Forest Grove Elder Services. Some are men; most are women; almost all are African American. With the assistance of wheelchairs, walkers, and canes, they slowly disembark from the Grove's fleet of vans. For some, the day is organized by bingo and crochet. For others, it is punctuated by medical exams and wound care. But no matter how differently the hours unfold, everyone's day will end in the same way: the Grove's vans will return everyone home. This is the promise of the Grove. No matter how sick or frail you might be, the Grove will do its best to keep you from the doors of the nursing home.

This is a difficult promise to keep. The Grove's members have all been certified by the state as having needs suitable for nursing home placement. Whether because of cognitive decline, physical disability, or medical complexity, everyone requires a significant amount of care. The resources available to provide this care are in short supply. All the Grove's members qualify for Medicaid, a marker of individual poverty and diminished family resources. The Grove's reliance on public payers is a sign of its own financial limitations in providing this care.

But provide this care it does. Teams of NPs, physicians, social workers, occupational therapists, RNs, physical therapists, and nursing aides all work in concert to provide the kind of comprehensive care that makes living in the community possible.[1] Each provider has specific expertise; however, caring for a high-needs population requires a level of coordination that does not happen spontaneously.

In most health care organizations, the person responsible for guiding group decisions is a physician. At the Grove, that person is a nurse practitioner.

"Ms. Payne. Can you think of anyone else who could come by a few times a day?"[2] Ms. Payne is eighty-six years old. Like most of the Grove's members, she lives with a litany of complaints: diabetes, arthritis, congestive heart failure. Yet none of these are why she is sitting in NP Michelle's office today.[3] In two weeks, Ms. Payne is scheduled to have cataract surgery to improve her increasingly cloudy vision. Michelle's aim is to make sure Ms. Payne is prepared for the operation. Cataract removal is a low-risk outpatient procedure, even for someone Ms. Payne's age. The surgery is not the problem. The problem is what will happen afterward.

I sit in the corner, trying to be unobtrusive in a room that seems full with three people. I listen as Michelle reviews the surgeon's postoperative instructions. Ms. Payne will need to apply a series of prescription eye drops—four times a day for four weeks—to control inflammation, prevent infection, and minimize complications. There is nothing remarkable about their application. One would simply stretch an arm upward, tilt one's head skyward, arch the arm over a selected eye, grip the bottle with a personal selection of fingers, then squeeze with the right amount of pressure. These coordinated steps, however, require a set of abilities that not everyone possesses. Ms. Payne has rheumatoid arthritis, a condition that not only inflames the joints but also often deforms them. This condition has left her hands curled in on themselves like talons. As Michelle describes how often the drops will need to be applied, all three of us look at these hands, our eyes filling with doubt.

Michelle begins to interrogate these doubts by testing what Ms. Payne can physically manage. She leaves the room and returns with a small plastic bottle that approximates the size and shape of the problematic eye drop container. She holds the bottle out to Ms. Payne and asks, "Do you think you can grasp it with your right hand?" Ms. Payne's right hand is the most visibly affected by her arthritis, but it is also her dominant hand. Ms. Payne looks at the bottle. She takes a few breaths before looking back at Michelle to say "No," with a note of finality. Michelle asks her to try with her left hand. Ms. Payne reaches out and successfully picks up the bottle. Following Michelle's prompts, she tries to reach her left arm over her head. But Ms. Payne's hand reaches its maximum height at just above shoulder level. She lowers her arm, shrugs her shoulders, and the encounter ends. Michelle's work, however, is just beginning.

After Ms. Payne leaves, Michelle confers with Claudia, the RN stationed across the hall, who assists Michelle and serves as her clinical sounding board. As they talk, I learn why Michelle did not mention what seems to be the most obvious solution: a home care aide. Every day, an army of aides takes medicine down from shelves, removes pillboxes from drawers, and helps people maneuver hard-to-open lids. What they do not do—at least not legally—is administer, or actively give, medication.[4] In everyday life, when we cannot administer our own medication, parents, children, even a good friend might be enlisted to assist. This practice is both common and legal as long as it is done for free, which explains why Michelle asks Ms. Payne whether she could think of anyone who might help. Anyone would have sufficed. However, when payment enters the equation, the universe of anyone shrinks considerably. In most states, only physicians and nurses can administer medication.[5] This includes prescription eye drops. The Grove would have had to pay for a much costlier RN to visit Ms. Payne four times a day, every day, for four weeks. Michelle knew without asking that the Grove was unlikely to approve such an expensive request.

Solving Ms. Payne's problem would require more than medical knowledge. It would require knowing how to navigate organizational systems both inside and outside the Grove. It would require gathering and using knowledge about Ms. Payne's resources. And it would involve knitting these disparate forms of knowledge together in a way that might be applied to the practical problem at hand. Over the next two weeks, I watch as Michelle performs this knitting together on Ms. Payne's behalf. She experiments with adaptive equipment that might make the task possible for Ms. Payne. When that is unsuccessful, she calls the surgeon—again and again until she gets a response—to see where the flexibility in the regimen might be. How frequently must the drops be given? Can they get away with three times a day over the weekend when the Grove is closed? Claudia meets with Ms. Payne separately to ask whether she is *sure* there isn't anyone who can assist her, even once a day. A cousin? A neighbor? Someone from her church? She reminds Ms. Payne, gently but firmly, that not wanting to ask is not the same thing as being unable to ask.

Michelle eventually crafts a plan that is one part neighbor, one part modified regime, and one part approval for two RN visits on weekends. Arriving at this complex calculus takes more than a little time and a great deal of work. The surgeon performs the technical miracle of curing the patient; Michelle performs a miracle of her own in helping to ensure the best possible outcome. With Ms. Payne's eyesight improved, the odds are good she will be able to stay in her own home for some time to come.

When I first arrived at the Grove, I was taken aback by the kind of intensive management that happened in its exam rooms. Very little of the activity in the clinic looked anything like what I expected to see within the medical encounter. But after months of observation, my initial surprise had settled into expectation. The case of Ms. Payne was not an outlier. Nor was Michelle an organizational aberration. The knitting together she performed for Ms. Payne was emblematic of the work of all the Grove's NPs—not only for patients undergoing low-risk surgeries but also for those living with end stage renal disease, struggling through the uncertainties of multiple sclerosis, or dying from cancer. After months of watching these NPs at work, I confess that I had started to take this state of affairs for granted: this was the work these NPs did; this was the work the Grove needed them to do. Michelle, however, may not have seen things in quite the same way. As we ended our last conversation about Ms. Payne, Michelle flashed a smile that was not really a smile and asked, "Now what part of all that was medical care?" Her question shook me out of my analytical complacency and, to a large extent, animates the questions at the heart of this account. How should we understand the care that NPs provide? And whose problems are they intended to solve?

From the ten-thousand-foot view of policy, the answers to both questions seem fairly clear. The care NPs provide should, ideally, be the same as that of physicians. Physician indignation notwithstanding, the scholarly consensus is that this is the case. Fifty years of research has demonstrated that patients who see NPs largely have the same outcomes as those who see physicians; when there is a discrepancy, it is usually in the NPs' favor (Buerhaus et al. 2018; DesRoches et al. 2017; Horrocks, Anderson, and Salisbury 2002; Landsperger et al. 2016; Laurant et al. 2004; Lenz et al. 2004; Martínez-González et al. 2014; Mundinger et al. 2000; Naylor and Kurtzman 2010; Newhouse et al. 2011; Ohman-Strickland et al. 2008; Ramsay, McKenzie, and Fish 1982; Stanik-Hutt et al. 2013). This robust evidence of equivalence grounds our collective assumptions about what NPs are for: to fill in for the missing physician.

Nurse practitioners were, in fact, intentionally created to deal with the growing scarcity of primary care physicians. In the 1960s, that scarcity was triggered by increased demand for services caused by the baby boom and the creation of public health insurance in the form of Medicare and Medicaid (Fairman 2008; Silver, Ford, and Steady 1967). Today, that scarcity is exacerbated by our aging population and the expansion of insurance through the Patient Protection and Affordable Care Act. Meeting this growing demand comes with a cost for insurers as well as health care organizations. That NPs are cheaper to train and less costly to employ than physicians has led to their being championed by policy makers and economists alike.

The NP as policy solution rests on a logic of substitution: when physicians cannot be found or afforded, the NP is a reasonable facsimile. The story of Ms. Payne suggests an alternate view of NP utility. Although paying for medical care remains an issue for many, it was not one for Ms. Payne. Like most Americans, she became eligible for Medicare when she reached the age of sixty-five. However, despite having a payer for medical services, she did not always have access to the full range of assistance she required. Ms. Payne needed help getting back and forth to medical interventions such as her cataract surgery. She needed help adhering to medical regimens such as her postoperative care instructions. Even before any of this practical work commenced, she needed someone to help her think through the help she needed and to coordinate with a range of people and organizations to make it happen. None of this assistance is paid for by Medicare because none of it qualifies as medical care. Even if she qualified for public or charitable programs to meet these needs, accessing and navigating those resources would require both knowledge and time. Although much has been made of the physician shortage, Ms. Payne's hurdles equally arose from the scarcity of supportive care.

Ms. Payne's story is also an illustration of the intertwined problems of economic and social precarity. Ms. Payne was not only a beneficiary of Medicare; she was also a recipient of Medicaid. Because poverty is the primary eligibility criterion for Medicaid, we often think of it as health care for the poor. However, it might be more accurate to call it long-term care for the disabled. While long-term care sometimes includes skilled nursing, it is primarily designed to assist with the activities of daily living, such as bathing, dressing, eating, and toileting. Because these services are excluded from Medicare, individuals and families have to pay for them on their own.

Few can shoulder these costs for years on end. In 2018, the yearly cost for forty hours a week of home care assistance was just under forty-six thousand dollars (Genworth 2018). These expenses are in addition to the mounting costs of medical care. Even the insured are expected to pay some portion of the costs of medications, hospitalizations, and provider visits. If nursing home placement becomes necessary, these costs can increase exponentially. In 2018, the annual cost of a semiprivate nursing home room was just over eighty-nine thousand dollars (Genworth 2018). While some may enter older adulthood in poverty, a great many others become poor as a consequence of failing health and mounting costs. For adults, it is often the combination of poverty and disability that results in eligibility for Medicaid.[6] As a consequence, Medicaid has become the single largest payer for long-term care in the US. In 2015, Medicaid paid for 36 percent of all home health care and 31.7 percent of all nursing home care (Burwell 2016).

Entering older adulthood intensifies not only economic needs but also social needs. In addition to paid care, most older adults rely on the unpaid assistance of family and friends (Freedman and Spillman 2014). Much of this assistance is material, such as help with transportation, grocery shopping, or household maintenance. Social support is also important. While aging itself does not increase social isolation, the illness and disability that often accompany it do (E. Y. Cornwell and Waite 2009a, 2009b; B. Cornwell, Laumann, and Schumm 2008). As one's needs increase, the resources in one's personal networks can become strained and sometimes exhausted. Medical vulnerability is often exacerbated by economic and social vulnerability, which in turn can negatively impact health and quality of life (Krause, Newsom, and Rook 2008; Newman 2003).

At the Grove, patients like Ms. Payne, faced with the interconnected problems of aging, illness, and poverty, turned to their NPs for a kind of work that was more than medical care. And at least some of the time, they found it. This book is an on-the-ground account of how a group of NPs cared for four hundred African American older adults living with poor health and limited economic resources. I followed these NPs as they saw patients, met with colleagues, and spoke with family. What I witnessed was less a facsimile of physician practices than a transformation of them. These NPs expanded the walls of the clinic to include not just medical complaints but a broad set of indigenous complaints. Patients presented with serious medical problems, such as congestive heart failure and diabetes, but they also brought a broader set of social and economic problems that, for them, were of equal importance. In response, the NPs practiced a professional openness to information and problems that are usually filtered out of the exam room. In response to this openness, patients and their families turned to the clinic as the place to get a diversity of needs met. Through this iterative cycle of openness and turning to, both the encounter and the work performed within it were transformed.

Clinic Work

The proposition that NPs are doing different work from physicians is grounded in a broader historical distinction between medicine and nursing. If physicians are the iconic providers of medical work, nurses are the iconic providers of care work. Broadly speaking, care work is defined as labor—paid and unpaid—that cares for members of society who cannot care for themselves because of age, illness, or disability (Duffy 2005; England 1992). While some scholars make further divisions between types of care work, what fundamentally distinguishes care work from other forms of labor is how it is performed and, often, who performs it (Duffy, Albelda, and Hammonds 2013; England 2005).[7]

Care work is based less on discrete services than on a general responsiveness to the needs of a person. In this way, care work is inherently relational. To use an example outside health care, kindergarten teachers are involved not just in educational instruction but in helping their charges eat, visit the toilet, and learn to socialize with one another. Moreover, how the work unfolds depends on the quality of the relationships that form between students, teachers, and parents. These features of the work cannot be separated from the fact that most care workers are women. Care work often overlaps with labor historically performed by women in the domestic sphere. Those who perform such work today continue to be marked by gender and the lower status associated with "women's work" (Charles and Grusky 2005; England 2010; England, Budig, and Folbre 2002). Despite the gendered devaluation that comes with seeing nursing as care work, nurses continue to claim care as a category and relationship as a feature that distinguishes the practice of nursing from the practice of medicine (Apesoa-Varano 2007, 2016; Evans 1996; Radwin 1996; Tanner et al. 1993).

In this account, I advance the notion of *clinic work* to illustrate the ways in which the Grove's NPs brought care work into the medical encounter. I employ this term for two reasons. First, it reflects the reality that the NPs' work was different in both form and content from the medical work of their physician colleagues. This difference was a consequence not of formal role distinctions but of a very different embodiment of what it meant to address patient complaints. When family disagreements and economic challenges were allowed to enter the clinic as part of the problem of disease management, what "disease management" meant was fundamentally altered. The observation of this difference came not only from me but also from the physicians—the providers best situated to evaluate what medical work was and was not. However, the NPs did address bodily complaints. Moreover, they were held to account by billing paperwork that required their work be made visible as medical work. Because they were doing this work from within the medical visit, this expansive form of clinic work had consequences not only for constructions of NP work but also for changing expectations of the medical encounter.

Second, I use clinic work to underline the ways in which the NPs' work invoked a different form of relationality—it was in deep relationship with the organization or clinic in which it was located. The Grove's NPs worked in a context organized around teams. The traditional boundaries one might draw between forms of expertise were less apparent in this organizational context. For patients whose problems were defined as much by poverty as by illness, and whose care was as much a feat of coordination as one of curative treatment, the lines between medical problems, social problems, and organizational problems were not easy to draw. In order to understand the construction of clinic work, I had to account for the ways in which some problems became NP problems while others did not. I discovered that the transformation of the clinic encounter was about neither the rearrangement of tasks nor the renegotiation of turf alone, but rather the working out of much deeper questions about what these problems were, and who was responsible for solving them. The organizational context in which this working out occurred is as much a part of the story as the providers themselves.

Organizational Care Work

Forest Grove Elder Services is not an ordinary outpatient clinic. It is a federally backed policy experiment to evaluate whether a comprehensive care model could ameliorate the state's economic burdens for long-term care. The pillars of the Grove's cost savings are coordination and capitation. The team model was its primary strategy for coordinating care. Each team consisted of a mandated mix of providers who worked together not only to provide direct medical, nursing, and supportive care but also to coordinate access to specialists, home care aides, and a host of ancillary services. To pay for this care, the Grove received monthly per capita or per member payments instead of fee-for-service reimbursements. This system provided an incentive to control costs and incentivized preventive over interventionist forms of care. Yet the Grove still operated under the quasi-market logic of all US health care: if its members did not believe they were receiving quality care, they could take their Medicaid and Medicare insurance elsewhere. The Grove had to provide not just cheaper care, but care of sufficient quality to successfully compete with other health care organizations.

In some ways, the Grove's experimental objective was to figure out how to deliver care work under the aegis of medical care. Its mission of intensive management and service coordination necessitated a layered understanding of each patient that required it to be responsive to a broad and variable set of individual needs. Even speaking of its patients as "members" was a nod to the expectation of relationship and responsibility. How does an organization—whose payment structure and regulatory environment still make it primarily accountable for medical work—deliver on the promise of providing the kind of patient-centered relationality required of care work?

At the Grove, the answer was through its NPs. One of the unique features of the Grove was that the NP, rather than the physician, was the formal head of the team. What it meant for the NPs to lead, however, was unclear. I observed that NP leadership was often reworked as NP responsibility. The NPs became solely responsible for ensuring that the Grove's mission of coordination was achieved. Within the expansive category of clinic work, the NPs were expected to deal with a broad set of problems not only as a way of helping their patients but also as a way of managing "difficult patients" for their employer. Doing so was not a simple matter. Various departments inside the Grove had to work together for member care, and the Grove had to communicate with a range of external organizations and family members. Moreover, the work of coordination seemed to generate as many problems as it solved. For the NPs, solving member problems often involved helping them navigate the inefficiencies of the organizations in which they sought care—including those at the Grove.

I argue that these NPs were not simply performing an expansive form of work on behalf of their patients; they were also providing an expansive form of *organizational care work* for their employer. As the NPs put out a range of social and organizational fires in the exam room, they were tasked with the invisible work of caring for the organization as they cared for patients. Clinic work was not in opposition to organizational demands but was partly constructed through the NPs' responsiveness to them. Problems not solved within the exam room became organizational problems. Patients whose social problems were significant hurdles to medical stability might transition to higher and more expensive forms of care. Members who struggled to navigate the Grove's inefficiencies might leave the program, expressing their dissatisfaction with the Grove in a way that was visible to the state. The NPs' performance of organizational care work made them a different kind of provider to patients, as well as a different kind of worker for their employer.

I entered the Grove attentive to the work of the NP. My main finding is that their labor became the primary means through which the Grove embodied its own mission of being a caring organization. How these NPs turned a broad set of concerns into clinic concerns reflected the expectations of their colleagues and employer as much as those of patients. I argue that these NPs were doing more than practicing medicine sprinkled with nurse-branded empathy; they were transforming the nature of the work itself.

Nursing's Utility under State Retrenchment

In exploring how these NPs solved problems for members and their employing organization, I had to grapple with the larger context in which these problems came into being. Physician scarcity is often treated as a naturally occurring problem inherent to developed countries with high demand for medical care. Yet this scarcity is not simply a consequence of consumer demand; it is a consequence of inequality. Not everyone struggles to find a physician; those with the least lucrative problems and the fewest resources are the most likely to have trouble accessing physician care. Perhaps one might wish that physicians would behave more altruistically. However, I argue that this uneven distribution of workers and work is a consequence of state inaction rather than individual career choices.

While the federal government has decried the physician shortage, it has largely taken a noninterventionist approach in addressing it. The state may coax or convince, but if physicians prefer dermatology to pediatrics, it will not compel. This reticence to use state power is not matched by a reticence to provide state funding. In 2015, the federal government provided 14.5 billion dollars to support medical residents working in teaching hospitals (Villagrana 2018). Even the economic disincentives to working in primary care are a function of state inattention. The comparative lucrativeness of specialty care is partly a consequence of unregulated prices. The federal government treats health care as a commodity and largely declines to interfere in the medical marketplace.

It becomes impossible to understand the creation of NPs without placing them within the context of what the state has decided *not* to do. In the years since I began this research, I have often been asked how NPs in the US compare to those in other parts of the world. The simple answer is that there is no other country that uses NPs in quite the same way. Governments that are less reluctant to directly control costs and personnel have less need for this new provider. Some countries, such as Canada, the United Kingdom, and Australia, are in the process of experimenting with NPs. Referencing the US as a model, they are deploying NPs to counter physician shortages in medically underserved areas. However, the NPs' extensive use and level of practice autonomy is a uniquely US phenomenon because the US is singular in having a hands-off approach to health care while largely financing its provision. In 2013, the federal government financed nearly two-thirds of all US health care (Himmelstein and Woolhandler 2016). In this context, the NP becomes a privatized, professional response to a set of policy problems that the state has declined to address through other means.

The pairing of state financing with privatized solutions has come to characterize not just health care policy but the US welfare state more broadly. Since the 1980s, the US has been the chief evangelist and implementor of neoliberal policy reforms (Centeno and Cohen 2012). Most of these reforms have been directed at deregulating money and labor; however, the general tenet of favoring markets over state influence has had a significant impact on social policy. A move toward smaller government has resulted in the downsizing and privatization of state and federal safety-net programs (Morgen 2001; Smith and Lipsky 2009). The socially and economically vulnerable have been the chief casualties of this approach. But there have also been professional ones.

Social workers were once the professional foot soldiers of the welfare state. In the early to mid-twentieth century, the robustness of professional social work reflected prevailing ideas about the state's role in addressing the symptoms and structural causes of poverty. As the government established relief programs and national efforts such as the War on Poverty, it relied on social workers to carry them out (Ehrenreich 1985). However, the use of state power to address inequality has fallen out of favor. Many of the programs that social workers once implemented have languished or disappeared. Those that remain are increasingly privatized, with social work's purview narrowed to policing client eligibility rather than providing therapeutic assistance or community development (Lipsky 1980; Schram and Silverman 2012; Smith and Lipsky 2009). With little to no state support, social work's professional decline was all but inevitable.

The story of social work's falling fortunes is more than just an interesting piece of occupational history. Its diminished status reflects the state's disavowal of any moral obligation to ameliorate social inequality. Although individual social workers continue to fight on behalf of their clients (Aronson and Smith 2010; Fabricant, Burghardt, and Epstein 2016), social work is in danger of becoming a disciplining agent of the state rather than the agent of social change its pioneers envisioned it to be (Schram and Silverman 2012; Soss, Fording, and Schram 2011). How this shift occurred is a question best addressed by historical analysis. But the logic of its reproduction can be understood through attention to the work that social workers do, and don't do, within the multidisciplinary environment of a health care organization.

The Grove was not unusual in employing NPs, but it was unusual in employing social workers. Social workers are a rarity in outpatient care because, usually, there is no payer for their work in this setting. At the Grove, social worker inclusion was required by the federal regulations that governed the program. Their presence raised an important question: How did the clinic encounter, rather than the social work encounter, come to be the appropriate location for the "sticky" problems of coordination and social precarity? I found that the social workers occupied a marginal position within an organization whose economic solvency was based on the performance of medical work. The logic of medical necessity that set priorities for the Grove's resources led to an institutional disinvestment in both the social workers and their realm of expertise. The social workers found that what they thought of as real social work had been replaced by labor that was largely in service to state-required paperwork and the regulatory requirements of medical work.

Comparing the plights of the Grove's NPs and its social workers revealed that the appearance of social problems in the exam room was a function not just of NP professional openness within the clinic encounter, but of the lack of resources given to address these problems outside it. The federal government has largely withdrawn itself as a payer for the problems of poverty even as its financing of medical care has soared. I argue that the saliency of the NP is as much a story of welfare state retrenchment as one of economic utility. The hurdles faced by the Grove's social workers illustrate the limitations of analyzing occupational strategies without placing them within a larger political economy.

The NP as policy solution is based on the logic of substitution. Once we start interrogating this logic, a new set of questions arises. As the sociologist Everett Hughes (1970) observed, experts do not just solve our problems; they shape our conceptions of them. The NP might be the kind of solution that rearranges the problem in new ways. Accordingly, the chapters that follow do more than describe the work of a particular category of clinician. They provide a view, from the ground up, of a broader reorganization of medical labor and its relationship to the ever-shifting division between medical problems and social problems. Nurse practitioners are often thought of as filling in for the absent physician. Together, these pages make the case that NPs are just as often filling in for the absent state.

The arguments I make in this book speak to broad changes in health care delivery. Although these arguments are far-reaching in their implications, they are made through the materiality of Forest Grove Elder Services. The first chapters of the book speak directly to the idea of NPs as a policy solution. In part I, I situate the Grove as both a professional and an organizational solution to the problems of health care, old age, and poverty. The Grove and its NPs do not exist in a vacuum; they coexist in a policy environment in which both nursing and health care organizations are seeking to capitalize on state support. I illustrate that the expansion of nursing's terrain is intertwined with changes in the organization and provision of care for older adults.

I then describe the professional resources that these NPs used to construct a notion of clinic work within this expanded terrain. In following the journey of member problems—how they are generated, to whom they are brought, and who fixes them—I reveal organizational logics about the type of expertise the Grove collectively believed resided within the clinic. Part of the work of this section is to reinterpret the clinical encounter as more than a meeting between a medical provider and the patient's chief complaint, but as an institutionally situated meeting of a range of complaints. I make the case for the NPs' performance of organizational care work by paying attention to the work they do and contrasting it with the work the physicians do not.

In part II, I demonstrate how the new notion of clinic work effectively reconstructs physician understandings of what constitutes medical work. I begin by looking directly at the relationship between NPs and physicians. The NPs I followed had three distinct views of who physicians were in relationship to their own practice: consultants, captains, or teammates. These three framings led to very different ways of being what each considered a competent NP. I then investigate how the physicians reoriented their own domain of work in the face of the NPs' view of their role. I pay particular attention to the unease experienced by physicians who found themselves working within NP-led teams, as well as how that unease was managed through actively relocating physician expertise outside the clinic. In doing so, I show that the NPs' clinic work was a relational concept that required adjustments in how physicians understood their own work.

In part III, I consider how the expansion of clinic work is inextricably tied to the shrinking domain of social work, both as a profession and as an orientation to social problems. Empirically, I ground my analysis in the everyday work of the Grove's social workers, who are positioned at the margins of an expanding clinic. I situate these observations within a broader view of social work's precarious professional position. Part of the challenge of claiming expertise for social work is its location in the devalued world of social problems. In this section, I argue that the legitimacy of the NP is related to the delegitimization of social work. The different fates of these two professions do not simply represent a problem of professional strategy; rather, they reflect an unwillingness, in policy and in ideology, to recognize the economic and political character of social problems. I end by questioning professionalization more generally as a privatized response to collective concerns.

Through illustrating these arguments, this book is both a meditation on and an empirical excavation of the possibilities NPs are forging within the confines of the medical encounter. When NPs fill the space that physicians have absented, they are embodying a different set of possibilities for what the health care encounter could be. In doing so, they are positioned to make visible not just the scarcity of physician labor but that of caring labor. Although sometimes self-conscious of the claim, nursing still relies on care as the bedrock of its professional identity and legitimacy. To care is not empty rhetoric; it is work. And although it is usually seen as ancillary to the main stage of medical interventions, health care organizations have never been more reliant on such work. The Grove's NPs may have been unique in the wealth of organizational resources available to them as they embodied nursing expertise. However, I believe they are not alone in being asked to solve different problems than their physician colleagues.

I suggest that, as providers with different professional experiences and held accountable to different expectations, NPs are opening the exam room to a different kind of clinical performance. Not only is this performance reshaping our ideas about medical work, but it is also a mirror that reflects how we choose to care for our most vulnerable citizens. In this account, I have avoided revisiting the question of what kind of work NPs should or should not do. Rather, I provide a closer look at the work they are actually doing, not just for their patients but for the health care organizations that employ them and for the state, which chooses to care in some ways but not others. In focusing on the work NPs do, I hope to both illuminate and trouble the relationship between who we think should solve our problems and what we understand those problems to be.

Part I

AN EXPANDED TERRAIN FOR NURSING

NURSING'S EXPERTISE

NP Francesca worked part-time in the Grove's clinic. The rest of her days were spent teaching nursing students. Before I had permission to begin observing in the clinic, one of the Grove's administrators encouraged me to meet with Francesca. Perhaps because she was an educator, the administrator believed Francesca would have "an interesting perspective on the Grove." Our meeting was scheduled at midday, when the clinic was closed for lunch. When I arrived at her office, I had a quick preview of the woman I was to meet. There was a sign on the door that read, "The Professor," in cursive font. Underneath was a picture of an owl who wore glasses and wielded an old-fashioned pointer. I cannot recall ever hearing anyone call her the Professor, but it was a name she had earned.

Francesca had received a PhD in gerontologic nursing research. She was not shy about describing herself as more academically than clinically oriented. By her own admission, doing the work of an NP was not her forte. She had taken the unusual route of getting her PhD before returning to school for the clinical NP master's degree. Along the way, she had developed a strong set of ideas about the work of an NP. I asked her, as I eventually asked all the NPs, to describe what being an NP meant. Her response was to take out a pen and teach.

"Medicine," she said, "sees the relationship between nursing and medicine like this." Francesca drew two circles: a large circle to represent medicine with a smaller circle for nursing contained inside it. "However, nursing has always argued that the relationship looks more like this." She then drew a second set of equal-sized circles that overlapped in the middle. Pointing to the right-hand circle, she said, "Medicine does many things that nurses can't do." As she pointed to the overlapping section, she continued, "And some of the things NPs do are also done by physicians." Then she pointed to the left-hand circle and said, "Yet nursing has things that only it does—knowledge that exists apart from medicine."

Francesca's sense of what nursing "has always argued" was informed by the long arc of nursing's history. But it was also shaped by her experience living through its more recent past. Francesca entered nursing as an RN in 1978. It was a time when neither nursing nor medicine was quite sure who NPs were. Nurses were initially wary of those who seemed to want to trade in their nursing identity for that of medicine (Fairman 2008). It was physician organizations, not nursing organizations, that initially welcomed NPs into the fold. This welcome, however, came with a risk. Physician organizations began arguing that NPs were no longer really nurses and therefore medicine, not nursing, should train and govern NPs (Fairman 2008).

The status and identity of the NP was not fully resolved until the mid-1980s. This period of uncertainty partly explains Francesca's somewhat circuitous route to becoming an NP. Nursing did eventually rally around NPs, so that today there is little question over which profession they belong to. However, Francesca's instruction underlines a reality that is often missing from debates about the NP: the boundary between the two professions is as important to nursing as it is to medicine. One of nursing's most enduring threats—to its identity, work, and governance—is that of being swallowed whole by medicine. To blur the line between them is to risk trading in nursing's diagram for medicine's, which shows nursing as a small island within the sea of medicine's domain. One of my primary claims is that NPs may be doing more than simply reproducing physician practices. That claim requires an understanding of the ways in which nursing's identity is grounded in assertions of difference, not interchangeability. In this chapter, I situate who the Grove's NPs understood themselves to be within nursing's larger political and existential fight for an identity apart from medicine.

A Profession Apart

Throughout the nineteenth century (and well into the twentieth), the family home was the site of most sick care in the US. Carried out as a woman's obligation to her family, nursing the sick was not viewed as something that required much in the way of knowledge or skill (Reverby 1987b). Whether a woman performed the work herself or discharged the duty to a servant, nursing work was akin to that of laundering clothes and scrubbing floors. The bonds of affection might imbue the work with deeper meaning, but as an activity, it was mere drudgery.

The story of how nursing transformed from drudgery into the work of a respected profession begins in the mid-1800s with the English reformer, Florence Nightingale. Nightingale has many accomplishments to her name, but she is widely known as the first person to make the case that nursing work required education (Reverby 1987a). She argued against the popular notion that women knew how to nurse by instinct or intuition; she believed potential nurses had to be both vetted and trained. Nightingale had an uphill battle. One of her primary challenges was the need to allay the fears of physicians and hospital administrators, who were suspicious of any new claimants to expertise over patient care. While navigating these more powerful actors was a daunting political hurdle, the cultural hurdle was just as formidable. In an era when even women of modest economic means did not work outside the home, Nightingale had to make the case that they could do so without losing their claims to respectability. Despite these hurdles, Nightingale's ideas came to fruition both in her native England and in the US.

There are several explanations for Nightingale's success, including savvy politicking. However, a key explanation lay in the decision to align her new ideas with preexisting ones. Similar to other female social reformers of the time, she made liberal use of a gendered, moral language to create a place for professional nursing (Ginzberg 1992; Kunzel 1995; Welter 1966). While members of the budding women's movement were beginning to argue that women should have some of the same rights as men, Nightingale's approach proved to be much more palatable. She argued for the extension of rights she believed women already held.

Nightingale drew heavily on the principle of separate spheres, a commonly accepted principle of the Victorian era. This principle held that women and men had fundamentally different natures that suited them for separate spheres of action: women were suited to the domestic, private sphere, while men were better suited to the public sphere. Nightingale contended that nursing was simply an extension of women's natural and rightful domain. Caring for the sick was already a woman's duty; she argued it could also be a woman's work (Nightingale 1860; Reverby 1987a). Nightingale's evocation of separate spheres quelled the fears of those who threatened to stand in nursing's way. Medicine would remain the province of men; women would work in their own, separate realm.[1]

Like most separate-but-equal doctrines, the principle of separate spheres was grounded in a deeper logic of inequality. The construction of nursing as a woman's profession would legitimate nursing's subordination to medicine for decades to come. The creation of a space apart, however, produced the possibility for nursing's autonomy and the construction of independent value. Nightingale was quite forthright in arguing that only nurses should control nursing work. Although noting that nurses had a duty to obey physicians in medical matters, she took great pains to argue for the necessity of separate chains of command (Holton 1984; Nightingale 1865). For Nightingale, nursing's autonomy was not just for the good of the nurse; it was for the good of the patient. She strongly believed that "medical therapeutics and 'curing' were of lesser importance to patient outcomes and she willingly left this realm to the physician" (Reverby 1987b, 7). In Nightingale's view, women were superior at nursing, and when it came to promoting health and well-being, nursing was superior to medicine (Holton 1984; Reverby 1987b). At a time when physicians were turning toward science and away from direct patient care, nursing began creating a corps of educated women whose distinct role was to observe patients, respond to their physical needs, and be attentive to their mental and social needs. Physicians would cure, but nurses would care—in a way that was skillful and that materially mattered for patients.

This initial framing set the nursing profession apart from medicine, with different work, different knowledge, and a different orientation to patient care. However, maintaining this separation has taken active work on the part of nursing. At different times and places, both hospitals and professional medicine have attempted to annex nurses into their own regimes (Fairman 2008; Reverby 1987a; Rosenberg 1995). Nursing, however, has been successful at preserving its own identity. In the US, twenty-first-century nursing maintains its own professional organizations, educates its own workers, and upholds autonomous standards for regulating its work. Nurses may not always have the same power as physicians, but they have taken pains to be neither absorbed nor governed by them.

The work of the NP might seem to be the breaking point of nursing's claims of separation from medicine. Nurse practitioners are licensed to provide the kind of care traditionally performed by physicians, such as assessing patients, making diagnoses, and providing or directing treatment. In twenty-two states and the District of Columbia, they can do so without physician oversight or involvement (American Association of Nurse Practitioners 2018). The NP's work and growing autonomy has arguably made the wall between medicine and nursing more porous than it has ever been. Nursing's original wariness of this new role illustrates the ways in which the NP was both an opportunity and a threat to internal notions of what it uniquely means to nurse (Barnes 2015; Brown and Olshansky 1998; Cusson and Strange 2008; Fairman 2008; Heitz, Steiner, and Burman 2004; Hill and Sawatzky 2011).

When I began my work on the NP, one of my first aims was to understand how the separation between medicine and nursing fared as NPs learned to, ostensibly, practice medicine. I turned my attention to a classic site of identity construction: professional schooling. In 2009, I spent twelve months following a cohort of NP students at Stanton School of Nursing. Stanton is highly ranked—what some might call elite. Elite schooling would not represent the modal experience; to be elite is defined by the status of being set apart. Elites are, however, usually the producers and chief circulators of group-level claims to legitimacy and status (Granfield 1992; Khan 2012; Reverby 1987a; Schleef 2006). If I wanted to understand how nursing fashioned and maintained an identity apart from medicine, elite schooling was one place to look.

The first thing I learned about nursing education is that from a credentialing perspective, every NP is a nurse. Prospective NPs must complete the education and licensure to become RNs before they can go on to train as NPs. When I spoke with Stanton's NP students about the transition from RN to NP, I expected to hear stories of "moving up" from nursing or of "getting through" the RN program as a credentialing hurdle. Instead, these students felt that the experience of being a nurse was fundamental to learning to be an NP (Trotter 2019). One student asserted that it was in being a nurse that he learned "to not just see the patient as a medical diagnosis or a set of problems," and that his experience as an RN gave him "a unique perspective on [providing] primary care as an NP." Another student shared: "It was in going through nursing school [and working as an RN] that I realized that nurses weren't just doctors' flunkies . . . that they were the ones at the bedside making a real difference in the patient's life." The time prospective NPs spent working at the bedside was not just about experience but about learning to embody what it meant to be a nurse. Even as they made their way through the NP curriculum, the salience of being a nurse remained.

To risk stating the obvious, it is not only RN education that happens in nursing schools but also NP education. Although ostensibly learning diagnostic medicine, these students were being taught a curriculum created by nurses and delivered by nursing faculty. Students were certainly cognizant that they were learning skills that, to some extent, still belonged to medicine. Yet they told stories that reframed much of this work as nursing work. Through educational narratives, they reworked nursing's traditional claims to "whole person care," "knowing the patient," and "relational interaction" (Apesoa-Varano 2016; Benner and Tanner 1987; Evans 1996; Radwin 1996; Tanner et al. 1993) into NP-specific modes of care (Trotter 2019).

It was at Stanton that I first began to realize that nursing's need to maintain its border with medicine was not only about professional control but also about claims to different expertise. Stanton's students were not learning how to be like physicians but were figuring out how to remain nurses. As nurses, they were called to be practitioners of care—not as an affective orientation but as an iconic form of care work marked by relationship and responsiveness (Duffy, Albelda, and Hammonds 2013; England 2005). Nursing's embodiment of care also invoked a different terrain of knowledge. I listened to faculty tell students, "doctors have their expertise, but you have your own." And I listened carefully as faculty and students narrated the location of that expertise: on the bodies of the socially vulnerable. These NPs in training were being told that their expertise lay in the very skills that medicine, in its turn toward specialization, had left behind. And that their utility was in serving those whom society had left behind: patients without health insurance, patients living in poverty, and patients struggling to manage their health under stressful circumstances. In Stanton's classrooms, the skills of relationship and of seeing the whole person put NPs in a position to be expert providers to those for whom economic and social precarity were daily realities. This was not simply a matter of empathy or compassion; it was about constructing a different kind of clinical problem to which they could apply nursing expertise (Trotter 2019).

I left Stanton with a firm sense of the kinds of stories, metaphors, and identities that NPs constructed to navigate their new role. At the same time, key questions remained about the relationship between what NPs said about themselves and how they might actually practice. The possibility that these were not one and the same was pointed out to me by a physician I knew who was completing a post-residency fellowship in pediatric anesthesiology. As I summarized my findings from Stanton, he countered, "Well, med students also form ideas about how they will practice. But then reality sets in." Indeed, what would happen when newly minted NPs brought their classroom-honed ideas to work—in a world not of their own making, but negotiated with the expectations of colleagues, employers, patients, and payers? To understand this more complex set of social processes, I would need to leave the nursing school.

There were any number of places I could have gone to see NPs at work. I could find NPs at a retail walk-in clinic, at a federally supported neighborhood health clinic, or at a high-end specialty practice. Faced with such diversity, I initially grasped at the idea of finding an average case. However, after months of conversations with Stanton faculty and students, I had already begun to doubt whether such a case existed. For providers whose role was in flux, organizational variation seemed to be more the rule than the exception (Fairman 2008). Students in particular had developed a belief that an organization's experience with NPs (and its physicians' attitudes toward them) was at least as important in shaping their work as the setting.

If I could not reliably find an average portrait of NP practice, I made it my mission to find one that was likely to represent nursing's ideal vision for NP practice. In the US, there is a group of health care organizations that self-identify as nurse-managed or nurse-led health care centers. Some are staffed by RNs trained in community or public health nursing while others provide NP-led primary care. But all embrace a vision of nursing leadership and, in agreement with the profession's larger claims, all assert their value in serving vulnerable populations and working to eliminate health disparities. Through a combination of word-of-mouth and organizational networks, I found what I believed to be all seven of such centers that provided primary care in one northeastern city. Each of these centers allowed me to spend an afternoon or two observing clinic operations and meet with at least one administrator, as well as the NPs. I learned about each organization's history, how it was financed, whom it served, and how it was staffed.

My goal in these conversations was both to develop an understanding of what being nurse managed meant and to investigate possibilities for fieldwork. This was how I found myself back in the halls of Stanton, speaking with the school's dean of community practice. Forest Grove Elder Services was on that list of seven because Stanton School of Nursing owned and operated it. Sitting across the desk from the dean, I described my broader research and my reason for wanting to add Forest Grove to my organizational tour. In response, she delivered what sounded like a warning: "The Grove is more than just a clinic." If I was looking for an ordinary clinic, the Grove was probably not where I wanted to be. She did, however, encourage me to visit the Grove, as an example of what nursing could and would do if allowed to embody its own orientation to patient care. I took both her warning and her encouragement to heart. Ultimately the Grove's uniqueness, rather than its representativeness, convinced me to stay for the next two and a half years.

The Grove was one of many policy experiments in community-based forms of long-term care. Its focus on comprehensive, coordinated care is fairly unique in a landscape dominated by piecemeal service provision. However, with a nursing school as its fiscal and administrative manager, the Grove was as much a demonstration of nursing leadership as an experiment in older adult care. For Stanton, the Grove was a stage upon which to elevate both the nursing profession and nursing work. While the Grove's model of care was not a nursing creation, Stanton often employed it as an exemplar of nursing expertise, professional mission, and nursing's utility to policy makers. As a nurse-managed organization, the Grove strove to embody a nursing approach to care even as it provided what patients and payers would recognize as medical care.

More than a Clinic

In 1998, Stanton opened the Grove with fewer than ten members. It was a humble operation, housed within a small, three-story storefront. Even with this modest start, Stanton knew it was potentially doing something big. Nursing does not have the same entrepreneurial history as medicine; its denizens have mostly been employees rather than owners. In a landscape where it remains uncommon for nurses to operate their own health care organizations, the Grove was an opportunity for Stanton to move nursing into new terrain. It was not long before they began having measurable success.

In less than five years, the Grove's member population had grown so large that it was able to open a second location. By 2005, membership had reached 250. The Grove was growing not just in size but in reputation. State and local politicians began to take notice of a program that seemed to appeal to consumers while also potentially lowering costs. In a nursing school newsletter, the dean of the nursing school reported that state administrators were asking the Grove to expand enough to accommodate five hundred members within the next two years. If the Grove wanted to continue growing, however, it would have to find a larger space.

Less than a mile from Stanton's campus stood a vacant building that seemed almost perfect. The building was four stories of chimney-red brick, containing over seventy thousand square feet of useable space. Not only was it large enough to consolidate the Grove's current members into one location, but it also had enough room to expand. The building seemed ideal in other ways. It had previously been a nursing home, giving it an optimal constellation of rooms and facilities to offer medical services, meals, and social activities. There was also a sense of poetic justice. Opening an alternative to institutional care on the grounds of a former nursing home seemed almost karmic; the building's story would eventually become a very satisfying one to tell. The space would also satisfy the needs of a growing organization.

In 2007, the Grove celebrated the grand opening of its new home. The move to a larger building was an aspirational one, not just for the organization but for the nursing school. Stanton was heavily invested in the Grove. The Grove's operating expenses were well over thirty-one million dollars, representing 40 percent of the nursing school's operating budget. Although it was one of several community practices that Stanton operated, the Grove's size and scope dwarfed the others, making it a unique and publicity-worthy achievement.

There were other ways in which the fortunes of Stanton and the Grove were intertwined. Stanton's nursing students routinely completed clinical rotations at the Grove. For its nursing faculty, the Grove was a common place to undertake gerontological nursing research. There were also links between Stanton and the NPs I followed: all but one was a Stanton graduate. If we assume that professional socialization is at least partly shaped by schooling, Stanton undoubtedly influenced these nurses' understanding of what it meant to be an NP (Becker et al. 1976; Fox 1957; Granfield 1992; Hafferty and Franks 1994). However, the ties between Stanton and the Grove were also about mission. In one Stanton newsletter, a board member was quoted as calling the Grove "an active personification" of what nursing stands for. The nursing school saw the Grove's focus on coordination and management as the organizational equivalent of nursing's own calls for relational, whole person care. For Stanton, the Grove was not just another clinic. It was a chance to showcase nursing's unique mission, leadership, and expertise.

Stanton's aim to elevate nursing work included the Grove's NPs. In and of itself, there is nothing particularly groundbreaking about employing NPs. However, the Grove was unique in placing the NP in a leadership role. While medical care was provided collaboratively by NPs and physicians, the NPs were explicitly named by Stanton as the leaders of the interdisciplinary teams and were, administratively, the primary care provider of record.[2] This naming is more revolutionary than it first appears.

Increasingly, teamwork in healthcare has been touted as a way to improve coordination, increase communication among providers, decrease medical errors, and ultimately, improve patient outcomes (Baker, Day, and Salas 2006; Institute of Medicine 2001; Rice 2000). However, critics have argued that the notion of teamwork is an illusion that masks entrenched forms of inequality (Apesoa-Varano and Varano 2014; Finn 2008; Finn, Learmonth, and Reedy 2010). Physician organizations require no such subterfuge. The American Medical Association (AMA) explicitly argues that the evocation of teams should not be employed as a leveling device; physicians should remain the rightful leaders in health care, teams or no teams (Permut 2016). At the Grove, however, this traditional hierarchy was turned on its head. In naming them as the principal providers in the clinic, Stanton gave the Grove's NPs an opening to reorder what care meant.

Nursing's Usefulness

If the Grove was an aspirational resource for Stanton, its NPs were on the front lines of nursing's continuing battle to prove its unique utility. However, at the level of clinical care, the Grove was also a testament to the contradictions of that utility. The first NPs were trained in pediatrics. Created to meet the demands of the baby boom, the pediatric NP was trained to provide "well child care." The expectation was that they would refer children with acute or chronic conditions to a physician (Silver, Ford, and Steady 1967). Popular accounts of NPs continue to stress their ability to provide "routine" care. Readers are asked to imagine yearly physicals, runny noses, and strep throat. Little, however, was routine about the Grove's members. No one knew that better than the NPs who cared for them.

When NP Norah first started working at the Grove, she was no novice. She had already been an NP for fifteen years. The last seven were spent at a retirement community. She knew older adults. She knew geriatric medicine. But when she first started treating the Grove's members, she recalls thinking, "Holy crap! These people are bad!" She had to learn how to manage conditions at a level of acuity she had rarely seen before. Norah was not alone. All the NPs I followed spoke about the challenges they faced in their first few years of working at the Grove. Not only were they seeing members living in complex circumstances, but as providers within a nursing home diversion program, they were also expected to stretch the limits of what is normally done in primary care. NP Anne, who had spent most of her career in acute care settings noted, "In a hospital, you refer everybody. Somebody's creatinine goes up with renal failure, you refer it to renal. You don't mess with it." At the Grove, things looked a little different. Anne continued, "You might bring them in. You might give them some fluids. Look at their med list. See if there's something you can cut back on." What Anne was describing is not primary care everywhere, but is often what it means to provide primary care for those with the highest burdens of disease and disability.

If the NPs' imagined patients are the vulnerable and underserved, the Grove was a place where the imagined came to life. Norah opined, "We're seeing people who just didn't have good health care throughout their lives." We know that poverty in particular and socioeconomic status in general play a significant role in determining health outcomes throughout the life course (Adler and Newman 2002; Braveman et al. 2005; Braveman, Egerter, and Williams 2011; Marmot 2004). There is increasing evidence that socioeconomic status continues to matter for health even in old age (Huguet, Kaplan, and Feeny 2008; Lyu and Burr 2016; Sudano and Baker 2006; Yao and Robert 2008, 2011). Because the Grove's members had to be medically frail or have significant cognitive deficits to qualify for enrollment, many had already borne years of costly medical interventions and home care expenses prior to coming to the Grove. These unrelenting economic stressors may have further worsened their health status.

Race was another factor that shaped the medical vulnerability of the Grove's members. In 2009, 96 percent of the Grove's members were African American. This was primarily by design. As a federal program, the Grove had a predefined catchment area of twelve zip codes. In seven of these areas, African Americans exceeded 70 percent of the population. Living as an African American in the US is itself a kind of medical vulnerability. There is a growing body of evidence to suggest that experiences of racial discrimination produce chronic stress that literally wears down the body, leading to premature aging and the early onset of chronic disease (Geronimus 1996; Geronimus et al. 2006; Williams 2012).

Nurse practitioners may have been created to provide routine care, but in becoming the providers of the poor, disabled, or otherwise medically marginalized, they have been asked to meet a fairly high bar of expertise (Buerhaus et al. 2018; DesRoches et al. 2017). Of course, they are not usually tasked with meeting this challenge alone. The vast majority of NPs work in a setting with some level of physician contribution (Health Resource and Services Administration 2014). This was particularly true at the Grove. In 2010, the Grove employed three full-time physicians and one part-time physician. In the Grove's state, NPs were required to establish a formal, documented relationship with a collaborating physician. The NP and MD signed written agreements that spelled out what the NP could and could not do. This formal performance of oversight, however, sometimes seemed to belie the level of independence expected of NPs in everyday practice.

At every other nurse-managed site I visited, the physicians were largely invisible. Once the collaborating agreement had been filed away, the physician's only responsibility was to be available for questions during the NP's practice hours—which usually translated to being available by telephone. These physicians had other jobs and had their own patients to see; acting as a collaborating physician was mainly a side gig. At five of the seven nurse-managed sites I visited, the physicians were not expected to ever appear in person. At the sixth site, the collaborating physician had a schedule for clinic visitations, but he came outside clinic hours to provide staff education, not to assist in patient care. The role of these collaborating physicians was to serve as a resource for the NPs, not for their patients.

This was not the situation at the Grove. The Grove's physicians did not have other jobs or other patients. The Grove was their full-time job, and they were expected to participate directly in patient care. This reality was partly a reflection of the Grove's organizational complexity. As a site within a larger federal program, the Grove had an additional layer of guidelines regarding physician presence. A physician was required to serve as medical director, and a physician was a required member of each interdisciplinary care team. The Grove may have been nurse managed, but it did not have the option of relegating physicians to the margins.

What all these physicians did on this stage of nursing excellence was one of the first questions I began asking at the Grove. Not everyone agreed upon the answer. One of the first people I asked was Katherine, who was trained as both a nurse and a social worker; at the Grove, her job was to plan and coordinate staff education. She said, "The nurse practitioners really do handle most of the care. We have physicians, but they are mostly consultants." I heard what she said, but I also heard how she said it. Even though we were alone in her office, she leaned in slightly and lowered her voice before she spoke these words, almost as if she were relaying a secret. I assumed what she was concealing was the role of the NPs. However, as I got to know the Grove better, I began wondering whether it was the role of the physicians she was trying to keep under wraps.

One of the initial formal interviews I completed was with the center's chief operating officer. I wanted to get her understanding of how the clinic was organized. She began by describing the roles of the NPs, the primary care nurses, and the wound care nurse. She then moved onto the appointment clerks, medical assistants, and the clinic receptionist. I listened patiently as she began to talk about the dental and podiatry services that the Grove provided in-house. For more than half an hour, she talked in great detail about the Grove's clinical services, but the word "physician" did not voluntarily come out of her mouth.

A similar silence around the physicians' role also seemed to pervade the clinic. In my first walk-through, I observed that outside each NP's office there was a printed list of clinical team members. The name of the full-time NP topped the list, followed by that of the part-time NP who supported the team. Then there was that of the primary care nurse and the team's medication nurse. The name of the home care coordinator and the home care nurse followed. The list ended with the name of the appointment clerk. There was no mention of the physicians.

The whispers, the silence, and the invisibility surrounding the physicians revealed a general unsettledness, not about the place of nursing but about that of medicine. In the world outside the Grove, it is the NP's scope of practice that is questioned. In that world, policy makers, insurers, nurses, and physicians continue to argue over just how independently NPs should be able to care for patients. But at the Grove, this question was turned on its head. In a nursing organization, crowded with nurses of all kinds, what exactly should the physicians be doing?

The Grove and its NPs were on the front lines of an enduring fight to both expand nursing's reach and maintain its separateness from medicine. While nursing has not been above marshaling claims of interchangeability when it appeals to policy makers, its advocates have also understood that its professional independence depends upon nursing maintaining work and knowledge that exist apart from medicine. The warning delivered by Stanton's dean was not just about the singularity of the Grove as a policy experiment; it was about the rarity of placing nursing's view of care at the center rather than at the periphery.

I chose to stay at the Grove because of what that rarity allowed me to see. In a site where nurses had more power to define their own work, I expected to see, in sharp relief, how NPs would embody professional difference from physicians while working in medicine's traditional domain. While much of the policy narrative has focused on how well the NP can approximate physician labor, I argue that it is their difference from, not likeness to, physicians that makes the NPs of particular utility to patients, health care organizations, and state policy makers.

FROM MEDICAL WORK TO CLINIC WORK

The Grove held morning meetings every day at eight forty-five a.m. Attendees would hear a rundown of which members had gone to the ER, who was being discharged from rehab, and who had died in the night. The meeting would begin with the on-call report. Outside business hours, there was a telephone number that members, families, and aides could use to relay questions and complaints. The on-call report was a summary of each call and how it had been handled. On most mornings, the reader of this report was NP Lori, one of the Grove's gero-psychiatric NPs. Once the meeting was called to order, she would stand, hold her notes in her right hand, and read.

"The home care nurse called to say that Allison Jones wasn't home yet. I believe she went on vacation."

NP Anne looked up when she heard Ms. Jones' name. She frowned and asked, "When was that? Because I went out last night to drop off medications."

"It was at . . ." Lori scanned through her notes to check ". . . five forty-five last night."

Anne continued frowning. "Hmm. Well. Okay," telegraphing through her voice that this was unlikely to be the end of the story.

"At six p.m., Mr. Simmons called needing wound supplies. I told the home care nurse. She is taking care of it."

Lori flipped the page on her notes and continued to read. "I got a call at ten p.m. Marlene Baker fell at home. I gave the message to Norah. She took care of it."

Without looking up from her notes, NP Norah confirmed, "It was taken care of."

"Stacey Ladner's son called. He was very angry. They sent a male caregiver to care for his mother last night. He wants a meeting." Anne interrupted to add, "It's not the first time this has happened. That's a grievance."

"The Gardens called. Arline Moore is not coming in today. She still has a cough and a sore throat." Lori looked up from her notes and suggested, "Nursing should go out to visit her soon. She hasn't been feeling well for a while." Lori addressed this suggestion to the room, but it was NP Michelle who wrote it down on her list of things to do.

"Denise Franks called about her meds. She had run out." Norah interjected, "But I took care of that. I took care of all of her meds." Lori shrugged. "Well, I called them in for the weekend. Maybe they didn't go through." Sometimes prescriptions did not go through, but Norah was certain that this had not happened with Ms. Franks. "I *know* her meds were taken care of. I personally tied them to her wheelchair before she left the center on Friday!"

On-call was the first item in a longer agenda. There were lists of which members had specialist appointments to attend, which members were requesting additional services, and whose families were lodging formal grievances. The daily reading of lists was an illustration of the complexity of caring for members whose problems appeared not just in exam rooms but in hospitals, nursing homes, assisted housing, and family homes. But morning meeting was more than an illustration of complex care provision; it was also a demonstration of how that care happened.

The principal actors in this daily performance were the NPs. And it was they who routinely disrupted this reading of facts. If there was a discrepancy between what they heard and what they knew, they would contest or amend what the organization believed to be true. While other attendees might voice a concern during the meeting, it was the NPs who actively performed the taking on of concerns. Even when they were silent, everyone could see them, seated collectively in the center of the room, responding to new information by making lists of their own. Through words, actions, and sheer presence, they performed their commitment to knowing about a wide range of member problems. Specialist appointments, problems with medication delivery—every piece of member-related information seemed to make it onto an NP's list. Moreover, this performance was a public one. Each NP's professional sense of responsibility was on display for the entire organization, from administrators to social workers to aides. We were there to witness what the NPs knew about their members and what they believed they needed to know. We also saw what they did with that information: they solved member problems.

In this chapter, I illustrate how this work unfolded, through attention to how certain problems arrived on the NPs' lists of things to do and how this arrival reflected both professional and organizational understandings of NP work. In an organization structured around teams, many people had access to member problems. From meetings to email exchanges, the NPs were joined by a host of others in receiving member information. This information was not only about disease processes but also about family relationships, community context, and each member's experience of the Grove's system of coordination. Yet I found that the NPs were singular in performing a professional openness to incorporating such diverse information into their clinical view of members.

The NPs' openness allowed them to cultivate a layered knowledge of each member that was distinct from the understandings of other providers on the team. More importantly, they were uniquely positioned to wield that knowledge from inside the medical encounter. In a health care context, problems that could be relocated to the clinic were treated with more urgency and more resources than those located outside the clinic. The act of relocating a broad range of problems to the medical encounter was at the core of the NPs' performance of what I call clinic work. The NPs were still responsible for treating and managing disease. However, their view of chief complaints was not limited to the biological body but extended to the socially and organizationally embedded body. Situated in the health care encounter, clinic work was not just added to traditional notions of medical work, it was a reconfiguration of what it meant to practice medicine . . . when it was practiced by nurses.

The Expanded Encounter

Norah was the full-time NP who anchored her team. In that role, she was responsible for the medical care of approximately one hundred members. When I first met her, I was struck by how closely she embodied my unarticulated ideal of a nurse. Demographically, she represents what nursing has looked like for most of its professional history: she is white, she is female, and she is a married mother of three. More than a confluence of demographic variables, Norah exuded a brand of easy confidence that one hopes to find at the bedside. "I'm good with people," she told me—not once, but several times. She made this pronouncement less as a boast than as a self-evident truth. "You've been here a while," she offered by way of explanation. "You know how I am." This confidence extended to her work. "I'm good at what I do. And I think the Grove appreciates that."

The Grove, it turned out, did appreciate Norah. If organizations can be thought of as having certain beliefs, the Grove believed that she was "one of the best" NPs.

I heard this assessment from the Grove's aides, its administrators, and more than a few of its clinicians. But what made Norah one of the best was not exactly transparent. The Grove, like many outpatient organizations, did not systematically analyze patient outcomes by provider. When I asked Norah to describe her understanding of how her work was assessed, she replied, "I don't think there's really much to do with—which is funny—performance." While there was some attention given to the timeliness of regulatory paperwork, the NPs were not held to account for chart audits or clinical benchmarks. Yet the Grove's sense of Norah's competence was not a mirage; it was grounded in the solidity of everyday experience. Norah was a problem solver. She seemed to take personal responsibility for attending to anything that stood between her members and improved health. For Norah, that meant expanding the terrain of the encounter beyond the walls of the exam room.

When I began following Norah, the first thing I noticed was the prominence of the telephone. Norah's day seemed to begin and end with attending to its demands. Each and every morning, she was greeted with the urgent blinking of the voice-mail light. These messages were almost exclusively from members and their families. There might be a call from Ms. Baker to report she had been up all night coughing. There might be a message from Ms. Joyner's daughter; when her mother returned home last night, her purse did not return with her. There might be a message from Mr. Rivers, who is concerned that his father has been acting strangely. Or from the triage nurse downstairs, who needs to notify Norah that a medication she was scheduled to administer has not arrived from the pharmacy.

In this more intimate version of the on-call report, Norah would repeat the same motions she had just performed in morning meeting: she would listen, and she would make decisions about what needed her attention. Norah's phone was not just a queuing device for when she was out of the office; it sounded out for attention throughout the day. The identity of these callers mirrored that of each morning's voice mails; they were usually members and their families. And more than anyone wished, these were often calls of complaint.

During one of my mornings with Norah, I sat behind her while she looked over her list of members for the day. When her phone rang, she answered with a swiftness that undoubtedly came with practice. "Oh hi, Carol." Carol is the daughter of one of Norah's members. Her mother was in a rehabilitation facility recovering from a hip fracture. Since her mother's needs were largely being taken care of at the facility, Carol had not called with a medical problem. She had called with a different kind of problem. The Grove had arranged to transport her mother from rehab to a follow-up appointment with the orthopedic surgeon.

However, no one at the Grove had notified the facility, and her mother was not ready for transport when the driver arrived. Consequently, her mother missed the appointment.

I listened as Norah made apologies to smooth over Carol's frustration, detailing what she would do to address the situation. "I'll have the [appointment clerk] reschedule the appointment. Next time, we'll make sure the nursing home knows." Norah wrote down this new item on the to-do list she keeps by her phone. When Norah said she'd contact the clerk, she meant that she would walk across the hall and speak directly to the clerk, verbally emphasizing how important it was to notify the nursing home "next time."

Before Norah could get through the pleasantries of ending the call, she noticed the clinic receptionist standing inside her doorway. During a routine vital sign check, Ms. Robins had presented with an elevated blood pressure. Per protocol, the receptionist came to alert Norah, asking, "Do you want to see her?" An elevated blood pressure is not always cause for immediate concern; some members have poorly controlled blood pressure, while others maintain a consistent blood pressure that runs higher than normal. Whether Norah chose to see Ms. Robins immediately was not solely dependent on the numbers, but on her particular clinical history.

Talking partly to herself and partly to us, Norah announced that Ms. Robins's pressure "is never elevated," and that yes, she would like to see her. Trying to be helpful, I volunteered to escort Ms. Robins from the waiting room to Norah's office. When I called her name, Ms. Robins arose under her own power. Without benefit of walker or cane, she walked slowly but easily beside me. Her physical abilities set her apart from much of the Grove's population. As we carried on a casual conversation about the center, I saw no evidence of impaired cognition. However, my assessment of her independence was misplaced. She was in fair physical health, but she had dementia, which made her an unreliable reporter of her own routines. Consequently, Norah did not begin the encounter by eliciting a history from Ms. Robins but by saying, "let's see if we can get your daughter on the phone."

Norah looked up the number in the electronic medical record and then dialed. Putting the call on speaker for Ms. Robins's benefit, she narrated her concern to the daughter and asked, "Has anything changed about her diet or her routine?" This simple question often elicits information about a caregiver's new job, a change in who resides with the member, or a new reliance on high-sodium frozen dinners. Today, Norah's questioning led to a simpler explanation for the elevated reading. According to the daughter, Ms. Robins had run out of blood pressure medication. As a comprehensive care organization, medication delivery was one of the things the Grove managed. Whatever had happened to Ms. Robins's medication was not the fault of an outside organization; it was the fault of the

Grove. Hiding her own exasperation, Norah confidently assured the daughter that the medication would go home with her mother today. This was not an empty promise. Norah did the work of making it a reality.

After ending the call, Norah turned to her computer and looked online at the pharmacy records. Finding those for Ms. Robins, she verified that the prescription was active and that the pharmacy did, indeed, fill it. Not content to trust the pharmacy's online system, Norah called the Grove's third-floor medication room to verify the order's receipt. Speaking directly with the medication nurse, she asked for confirmation that Ms. Robins's medication refills would go home with her on the van this afternoon. Before she hung up, she made a final request to the med room nurse: "Can you come down and give [Ms. Robins] her regular dose of Lasix [a blood pressure medication]? She missed it this morning."

The traditional medical encounter does not usually contain these kinds of problems. An assumed part of diagnostic thinking requires filtering a patient's diverse complaints until a singular, medically defined complaint remains. For Norah, the problem, and therefore the solution, was more complicated than just what the body was doing. Instead of a winnowing out of members' indigenous complaints, she expanded the encounter to include them. Addressing the problem meant helping members gain access to the right specialists for a successful recovery. It meant dealing with the everyday difficulties of medication compliance. She expanded the encounter to include family members—using the phone to dissolve the time and distance between the clinic and what was happening at home or rehab. She organized the action of the Grove's institutional caregivers such as the medication nurses, the appointment clerks, and the transportation department. And just as importantly, she often smoothed over the frustrations of members and their families, not by managing their emotions but by taking responsibility for their problems.

For Norah, there was no contradiction between the work she performed and her ideas about what NPs do. When I asked Norah to describe the NPs' approach to patient care, she responded, "The nursing model is much more holistic [than the medical model]. You're looking at the whole person. Yes, disease is part of the person, but so is their environment, so is their mentation, their spirit, so is their social environment. So I think instinctually we all—nurses—that's how we look at some things." This professional orientation informed how she described the role of the NP at the Grove. Norah described the NPs as "like the air traffic controller of the members and their needs." Although each team contained a range of providers, she believed that the NPs were best positioned to "hear things or identify [member] needs." For Norah, this positioning was not an individual orientation but a professional one. "NPs have really taken on that kind of responsibility. *It's the nature of the profession.*"

Norah may have been considered an exemplar of NP skill, but she was not unique in expressing her belief that NPs had a distinct professional approach. NP Alice was one of the Grove's part-time NPs. She did not have her own team; she saw members in support of the work of a full-time NP. When I asked her to describe her role at the Grove, she replied, "I'm the gatekeeper that sends things out, but yet I also try to manage [members'] medicines and overall health. That's my 'big picture.' But I'm also trying to coordinate all of the ancillary and other people that help me keep them functional. My job is to keep them as functional as long as possible. And that's what I do."

Similarly to Norah, Alice went on to contrast this orientation to that of the medical model that physicians employed. "Of course a doctor would tell you they do that too. But again, I doubt that they're going to check to see what the dentist had to say or what the optometrist had to say. Lots of times they don't even really—they don't listen well." It is notable that this was the experience of a part-time NP. Even though the patients she saw were not, in an organizational sense, "her members," Alice's understanding of what NPs do nonetheless shaped her sense of responsibility. Sometimes that care looked similar to that of the physician—for example, managing medicines and making referrals. But sometimes that work was in an arena that Alice put into the exclusive purview of nursing. From the vantage point of the NPs, listening well to members was one of the core ideals of what it meant to be a good provider. Listening well took skill. It also took time.

Michelle was another full-time NP with her own panel of members. One afternoon, I sat with her as she met with Mr. George. She was meeting with him because his weight had gone up by seven pounds in less than two weeks. She needed to figure out why. Mr. George had congestive heart failure. Rapid weight gain from fluid retention is one of the classic signs that something is amiss. It could be a worsening of his heart; it could be a change in his diet; it could be a problem with his medication. This was the kind of slow-moving emergency that the Grove's NPs faced on a daily basis. If Mr. George retained too much fluid, it might eventually move to his lungs. If Michelle could not figure out the problem fairly quickly, he might find himself struggling to breathe.

Michelle often employed a style that could best be described as playing dumb. When she wanted to understand a problem, either from a member, family, or staff, she asked questions that seemed to conceal what she believed she already knew. I watched as Michelle spent half an hour listening to Mr. George describe how he took his medications and when. She was meticulous in her questioning. Because Mr. George was not conversant with the names of the medications he took, she showed him pictures of each of his pills as she asked him when he took them. Her questions were open-ended. Therefore, along with hearing the information she may have been interested in, she also heard what Mr. George was interested in. He had his own ideas about how each of the medications made him feel. He asked questions of his own about why he was taking certain pills or why the pharmacy had switched him from brand name drugs to generics. When Michelle got to one of his last medications, he said, "This one I take halfways." She stopped and asked, "What do you mean by halfways?" After a bit of questioning, Michelle learned that Mr. George was only taking half this pill; he was concerned about side effects and believed he felt better when he took less of it. He did not know that the pill he was taking less of was the medication that helped him manage his heart failure.

At the Grove, the expansion of the clinic encounter required a professional openness to information from inside the exam room as well as from outside it. Michelle learned a lot about Mr. George in this interaction. She learned how he reasoned about which pills to take and when. She learned that despite not knowing which pills were for which condition, he was otherwise willing and compliant with taking his medications. She learned more about his relationship with a neighbor who sometimes came over to help him put groceries away. And she also learned why Mr. George was retaining fluid.

The Epistemology of Professional Openness

The position of leaving oneself open is in accordance with the stories nursing tells about itself. Scholarship on nursing practices has identified "whole person care," "knowing the patient," and "relational interaction" as unique to nursing forms of care (Apesoa-Varano 2016; Benner and Tanner 1987; Evans 1996; Radwin 1996; Tanner et al. 1993). Some nursing scholars have raised questions about the utility of grounding nursing identity in a rhetoric of care rather than in knowledge or technical know-how (Allen 2004; Dingwall and Allen 2001; Gordon and Nelson 2006; Nelson and Gordon 2006). Nursing, they argue, will never get its due as long as it is associated with ephemeral qualities rather than concrete skills. In spite of the arguments of professional advocates, care remains salient to practicing nurses and continues to ground an identity that distinguishes their work from that of physicians (Apesoa-Varano 2007).

Maintaining a separate identity is serious business. Nursing's claims to its own expertise have been key both to its early formation and to ongoing group cohesion (Fairman 2008; Reverby 1987a). These claims continue to matter; they provide the cultural tools for NPs to forge not only a different kind of medical career but also different notions of the medical encounter. When I interviewed Stanton's NP students, they uniformly spoke of a nursing model of care as separate and distinct from the medical model. When I asked them what it means to care for patients as NPs rather than as physicians, they distinguished nursing from medicine with phrases such as "holistic," "whole person care," "relationship-based," and "not just seeing the patient as a medical diagnosis." Even as they explicitly noted that becoming NPs required them to learn new skills from medicine, they had a persistent belief that as NPs, they would be employing these skills "like nurses" rather than "like physicians" (Trotter 2019). These were not just the sentiments of untried students; they were mirrored in the words of NPs on Stanton's faculty who had decades of experience.

Nursing may claim NP difference; however, we know very little about how such claims are embodied (or not) in the clinical encounter.[1] By contrast, we know a great deal about the structure of physician-led encounters. Instead of professional openness, physician encounters are marked by control (Mishler 1985; Waitzkin 1989). While there is conversation between patient and provider, the rhythm and cadence of the encounter is governed by the physician (Frankel 1990; J. Katz 1984; West 1984). The physician asks questions of the patient as well as the physical body, through tests and examinations. Through this questioning, the physician shapes the meaning of the encounter. Patients may come with their own understandings of their problems, but the goal of the physician is to construct a medical narrative out of patient accounts. This is the core of the physician's job: to tame chaotic and sometimes contradictory pieces of information into an orderly diagnosis. While some scholars have critiqued the systematic removal of patient experience and meaning during the medical exam (Mishler 1985), a chief reason why patients seek physician counsel is to be offered a distinctly medical explanation for their individual suffering (Freidson 1988b). The power dynamic between them may be asymmetric, but patients and physicians enact a largely shared expectation of both the encounter and the role that each will play.

As a sociologist and a patient, this is the rubric of the medical encounter I brought with me to the Grove. Yet I observed that the NPs' encounters were seemingly controlled as much by the members as by the NPs. I found that members were able to assert the urgency of their own needs through the logic of medical necessity. Even though the Grove is an outpatient organization, the assumption of medical acuity legitimated access to most of its resources. At a fundamental level, medical need was used to triage access to the center. Member attendance schedules varied between one and five days a week. While these schedules were sometimes based on member choice, determinations of medical necessity were used to limit attendance. Socialization and well-being were assessed as part of the members' needs, but medical necessity was the primary argument that justified center attendance. This logic was similarly used to prioritize access to services within the center. Any of the center's social activities could be supplanted by medical need. Members might be asked to interrupt Bible study or a musical performance in order to meet with an NP or the wound care nurse. The Grove did its best to accommodate member preferences, but primacy was given to clinic-based services. This primacy was not, however, only a logic that was imposed on members; it was often a logic that members employed.

Members actively used this logic for their own purposes. The Grove's aides were not always able to stop what they were doing to accede to requests to be taken to the first floor for bingo, but a request to go to the clinic was rarely ignored. This open-door policy created a clinic that was as much a member space as a clinician space. Members would enter the clinic with problems ranging from chest pains to constipation. They would come in to complain that they had missed lunch because they were out on an appointment and got back to the center late. Sometimes, they came to share a picture of a grandchild or to enjoy the relative quiet of the waiting room. The Grove's members made their own use of clinic resources.

Not everyone was supportive of this expansive use of the clinic. There was an unresolved tension between meeting the needs of members and getting the clinic to operate more like a standard medical office. But the NPs were reluctant to limit member access to their attentions. The defining feature of the Grove's members was not age but illness. As one administrator noted, "these people can turn on a dime." For the NPs, this medical complexity was inextricable from an individual's social context. Norah opined, "It's one thing if we're all making a widget and it's supposed to look the same way over and over again. But when you're dealing with human beings, there's so many other elements involved." The NPs sometimes complained about their "frequent flyers," but their doors remained open nonetheless. From the perspective of the members, this openness worked out in their favor. The clinic was the one part of the center where every member was guaranteed a face-to-face conversation.

The logic of medical necessity kept the doors of the clinic open. When members arrived, they found a matching level of openness among the NPs. This openness effectively expanded the walls of the clinic, creating not just more frequent encounters, but also encounters distributed across time and space. The NPs not only saw members in exam rooms; they took calls and voice-mail messages directly from members and families. They initiated their own calls to providers both within and without the Grove. They even did short consultations in hallways and waiting rooms. The Grove's clinic was embedded within the larger day center. Any time an NP left her office, she found herself interacting with member needs. In addition to a few sociable "good mornings," any NP who entered the waiting room might hear someone call out, "Michelle!" or "Norah!" "All I need is Lantus [a brand of insulin]. I'm out!" If their issues could be addressed with a few short questions, the NPs were often inclined to act rather than wait. But being responsive to members and their families was only half of clinic work. The other half was being responsive to staff.

Caring for the Organization

While members and their families relied on the telephone to communicate with the NPs, their colleagues relied on email. Some emails were sent to individuals, but almost all member-related emails were addressed to the team. When I first began observing in the clinic, Norah asked me, "Are you on the team email lists? If you're not, you have to be. You won't understand how we work unless you're on team email." About her own team, Norah noted, "We solve a lot of our problems by email. I think that's partly what makes us so efficient. We come to an agreement about things without formal, scheduled meetings."

Whether email improved team efficiency was up for debate, but it was undisputedly the Grove's primary way of communicating about members. The implicit purpose of sending these emails was not just to share information but to spur some kind of action; someone had identified a member problem that the team needed to solve. Even when the sender of an email addressed a communication to a specific person, it was common practice to cc the entire team. In theory, each clinician would evaluate which emails belonged to his or her domain of expertise. In practice, the question of appropriate expertise was unclear. Because the Grove was a comprehensive care organization, the problems it addressed rarely fit discretely into a single category. Who addressed a concern often seemed less a matter of licensure and more a matter of who took responsibility. Moreover, given the prominence of email, this taking on of responsibility was publicly performed. Not only team-based clinicians were on each email list but also administrators, supervisors, and direct care workers who worked across teams. In this public arena, when problems were handed off to the team, it was the NPs who often responded.

If checking voice mails was the first thing the NPs did each morning, checking emails was the second. One morning, I watched as Anne scanned through her team emails. One of those messages was about Ms. Tyne, who was being discharged from the hospital to home that morning. There was already an organizationally defined chain of events that happened when a member left the hospital, starting with the member being brought to the center to be seen by an NP. This chain of events was defined by protocol; the email sent to the team was not intended to start a conversation, but as an FYI. However, for Anne, there was a more immediate response required.

Less than half an hour prior, Anne had listened to the reading of member appointments in morning meeting. In paying attention to this list, she possessed information that might solve a problem that had not yet surfaced. Anne sent an email to transportation, cc'ing her question to the team: "Is it still possible for Ms. Tyne to get to her neurology appointment this afternoon? It took us months to get her that appointment." Minutes later, she got a response from transportation: "We'll see what we can do." The team may have been the recipient of this information, but it was Anne who had the knowledge to respond. More importantly, she responded quickly enough that a potential problem was avoided.

At other times, emails were sent to the team with a defined problem. One afternoon, Michelle received an email concerning Ms. Violet. That morning, Ms. Violet had presented with symptoms of a possible retinal detachment. Unless addressed quickly, this condition can permanently impair vision. Michelle had completed the referral paperwork for an urgent visit with the ophthalmologist and had arranged transportation through the Grove. A few hours later, Michelle received a team email from transportation saying, "Ms. Violet has declined transportation. She said she doesn't want to go and sit around all day."

Individuals do have the right to refuse medical care. The Grove's members had that right as well. However, the Grove's providers could not always take such refusals at face value. Their members had varying levels of medical literacy; some might not clearly understand the implications of their refusal. There was also the possibility of dementia-related confusion. Some members might very well have forgotten why they were going to an appointment in the first place. This was the kind of uncertainty that made Michelle leave her office in search of Ms. Violet. She found her in the first-floor dining room. She sat down next to her and explained the urgency of the appointment. Michelle relayed the dangers more directly than she had before. "Do you want to take the risk of going blind? That's what can happen." Apprised of the potential seriousness of her symptoms, Ms. Violet agreed to go. Michelle returned to her office and called transportation. "The appointment," she told them, "is back on."

With the same urgency that drove their responses to calls from daughters and sons, the NPs responded to the concerns of their colleagues. Acting as the air traffic controllers of members' needs, they read emails from transportation, notifying them that Mr. Wells refused to get on the van that morning; from the home care nurse, noting that Ms. Brown's blood sugar was over two hundred; or from a home care aide who observed that Ms. Lawrence's refrigerator was stockpiled with months' worth of unused insulin. Everyone on the team received these emails, but if it seemed a matter of medical necessity, the NP took up the concern. In a population as acutely ill as the Grove's, it seemed that almost anything could qualify as a medical necessity. And it was to almost anything that the NPs seemed to respond.

For many of the Grove's staff, the NPs' responsiveness was highly valued. One of the appointment clerks expressed this quality as belonging uniquely to the NPs. "If I need my nurse practitioner, I know where she is. Any four of them, I know where they are. You know? If I need something, it's done. And if they need something, they know it's done." She compared the NPs to the physicians in saying, "These nurse practitioners? They do some really amazing things. I guess it's the regulation that you have to have a doctor here. Okay, fine. But sometimes nurse practitioners are much better than doctors." The clerk was not equipped to assess clinical effectiveness. She knew, however, what "better" meant for her. "Better" was being available. This availability was partly about being physically located in the clinic. But it also described an existential openness to recategorizing a broad range of concerns as clinic concerns such that if a member—or a clerk—needed something, "it's done." The NPs' openness encompassed all member problems, whether they were presented by members or by staff.

The clerk's words also conveyed reciprocity. If the clerk needed something, she could count on the NPs. But if they needed something from her, she was there. This reciprocity created possibilities for information sharing. The primary job of each team's clerk was to make and organize outside appointments for members. This entailed more than just calling the rheumatologist or endocrinologist to set up the appointment. The clerks were responsible for organizing all the small but crucial details that made the appointment possible. They had to coordinate with transportation over both the time and the necessary assistance required. They faxed over preliminary test results. They called to remind members and family caregivers of the appointment, explain the travel details, and to emphasize any required preparation, such as fasting.

These were the components of the job, but in order to do the job well, the clerks had to perform their own form of social triage. A good clerk knew that Mr. Scheller always missed early morning appointments. A good clerk knew which adult child or neighbor needed to be called to help Ms. Taylor remember that she had an appointment on Wednesday. A good clerk knew which members needed a few extra phone calls and some direct encouragement to get to medical appointments. The importance of this information may have explained why the NPs took on the responsibility of discussing appointments with their clerks— either through email or direct conversation—on a weekly basis. It was during these conversations that an NP had the opportunity to learn the kinds of things that a good clerk knows.

Anne was an NP who preferred face-to-face discussions with her clerk. On any given Monday, Anne might pick up the phone and call her clerk. "Stacey? Can we talk about appointments?" On one such Monday, Stacey responded by appearing in Anne's doorway. "Well," Stacey began, "Mr. Fromm has a derm appointment. He already said he's not going." "What's the appointment for?" Stacy shrugged her shoulders. Anne looked up the request for consult in the medical records and read aloud, "'Mole on left temple.' Okay. Well, whatever it is, it's not urgent and he doesn't want to go. Cancel the appointment." The two of them don't discuss every appointment, just the ones Anne has questions about. Including Ms. Stoke's colonoscopy. "Have we made arrangements for an aide to go with her?" Ms. Stokes had no family in the city. She also struggled with anxiety. Without someone to go with her, she might not go through with the procedure. Stacey asked Anne, "Do you think she needs anything else? For the anxiety?" Anne considered before answering, "I think she'll be okay with an aide."

The clerks might not always know which appointments were medically crucial, but the NPs might not always know which collection of resources would be needed to get a member to an appointment. These conversations between the clerks and the NPs provided an opportunity not just for the NP to share her clinical knowledge with the clerk, but for the clerk to share information with the NP. Both learned something in the exchange. What the NPs learned was ever-more-detailed information about the lives of their members. And they learned it not only by listening to complaints from members and their families but also by leaving their doors open to an endless stream of clerks, RNs, and aides. This information, too, became part of the expanded clinical encounter.

When I first witnessed the rhythms of each NP's day, I characterized them as beset with interruptions. I saw the phone calls, emails, and doorway visitations as intrusions on the "real" medical encounters I expected to see. One of my initial thoughts was that the NPs inhabited a slightly updated portrait of the harried floor nurse—called to be responsive to everyone and everything with little authority to say no. As I discuss in later chapters, there is an element of this explanation that rings true. But I also began to understand that the NPs were not just "doing everything." In leaving themselves open to member information, they were cultivating expertise.

Cultivating Expertise

Each of the NPs had the support of an RN in a role the Grove called the primary care nurse. One such nurse summed up her role as "a lot of computer work" in creating care plans for the members, doing patient education, assisting with wound care, and calling members at home to remind them about medications or just to "check in" if the nurse decided that would be beneficial. The NPs had a much more evocative way of describing the primary care nurse. For Anne, her primary care nurse was "like my right arm." This was particularly true for the primary care nurse who worked with Norah. RN Joanne's office was right across the narrow hallway from Norah's. With their doorways facing one another, they could sit at their respective desks and hold entire conversations throughout the day. Norah had a penchant for annotating her activities aloud. "Joanne!" she might call out while doing billing paperwork. "Ms. Carnissi has twenty-one [billable] problems!" From these conversations, Joanne came to know much of what Norah knew about their members. But she also developed an understanding of what it meant to do the work of an NP.

In spending time with Joanne, I learned that she was currently taking classes for a master's degree in business. She did not want to do the work of an RN for the rest of her life. I asked, "Why business? Why not become an NP of some kind?" she answered from the perspective of someone who had watched Norah's work for almost two years. "The NPs do the work. They do all the hard work." When I asked what the hard work was, she responded, "Let's say you're Mr. Smith. And you're in the hospital right now. And you call one of our doctors. Chances are, they don't know Mr. Smith like an NP knows Mr. Smith: his family situation, including his financial situation; what's going on, what hospital work we've done in the past; what has worked for him in the past." Joanne marshaled her own empirical data to back up this claim.

> You pull a physician note [from the medical record] and it's empty. Not empty, but there's nothing in there but, you know, a few words. It's like, 'oh, yeah, I've seen them; they're fine.' But you have the NP notes going much deeper into what is found. You find the situation and the conditions of daily living because they're coming in from their nursing background when you access all those things that you're adding it to the problem. It's more holistic, you know. The physician goes, 'oh, no chest pain today' . . . and that's it. . . . The physician's notes sometimes lack that personal touch to it where you can tell that they do not have the connections with people that the NPs have.

From Joanne's perspective, the hard work that the NPs performed gave them a better relationship with the members, which in turn gave them a better understanding of members. I pondered Joanne's words for some time. To speak of relationship is usually to invoke the intangible world of emotions. Nursing's own claim as a caring profession is itself evocative of the realm of feelings. Yet when Joanne illustrated this term, she did not describe an affective tie between NP and member, but one born of a deep, layered knowledge of patients. Moreover, she was explicit in calling out the material action required to cultivate that knowledge. For Joanne, this was not the result of an emotional attachment; it was the result of hard work.

It was not, however, always easy to see how this work got done. There was nothing inherent to the NPs' organizational position that gave them access to more or better information about members. The NPs were firmly ensconced in the clinic; although some of the Grove's staff did visit member homes, the NPs did not routinely do so. Neither did their days, structured by nine-to-five clinic hours, encourage family member visits. The Grove's medical director was not shy about describing this as a shortcoming in the way the NPs practiced. From her own experience as a physician in community-based practice, she believed that the NPs needed to have more face-to-face meetings with family if they wanted to build relationships and include them in clinical decision-making. However, the NPs' view of their members was not as truncated as the medical director believed.

From inside the clinic, the NPs gathered this information from members and their families through patient exams, telephone calls, and emails from administrators and clinical staff, as well as from support and caregiving staff through direct conversation. The NPs often had the most complete picture of their members, not just because of what they were privy to inside the medical encounter but because of the ways in which they expanded the encounter to include the view from outside it. They could describe the basic layouts of member homes or the contents of a refrigerator, and knew whether a neighbor could be called on in a pinch. They knew who lived alone, who had a difficult sister, and who would never remember to reorder their meds. Acquiring information about members was not a passive activity. It required an openness to sources usually excluded from the medical encounter. In my observations, these NPs gathered such information not in spite of, but because of, their expansion of the clinical encounter.

Like Joanne, I also witnessed the NPs doing the "hard work" in the clinic. But hard work is not quite the same thing as expert work. It would be tempting to conclude that the NPs were enacting a division of labor in which the physicians did the traditional work of making medical decisions while the NPs did a somewhat expanded version of bedside nursing work: dispensing medications, attending to bodily needs, and monitoring patients. This way of dividing up the work would be in keeping with the traditional boundary between nursing and medicine. As is seen in later chapters, the Grove's physicians and NPs did perform different work. Yet the border that separated their activities did not align so neatly with formal occupational distinctions. In part, both administrative and clinical logics constrained the embodiment of nursing difference in the primary care exam room.

Despite being a nurse-managed organization, the Grove did not have the option of moving traditional nursing work from periphery to center. The core reason for this limitation was financial. For any health care organization that relies on third-party payment, what counts as medical work is not a matter of ideology but of the predefined rules of reimbursement. Under these constraints, the Grove had to economically justify NP work. In the case of the Grove, whose funding came from Medicaid and Medicare, the cost of the entire operation, from recreational activities to physical therapy, was legitimated by the documented, reimbursable medical activities that happened inside the clinic. "Whether we like it or not," explained Norah, "it's all about the money. Really, we can't function unless the money comes through. If [the NPs] don't do our part of it and make sure the money comes through, then it's an issue."

Making sure "the money comes through" meant attending to encounters that resulted in new or updated billing codes such as enrolling new patients, documenting new diagnoses, or correctly identifying the worsening of old ones. Billing codes are what determine what an insurer will pay for a visit or procedure. Even under the Grove's capitation system, these codes were part of the algorithm that determined patient acuity, which was directly tied to the per capita rate the Grove received. The Grove was also mandated to complete comprehensive assessments that included an in-person medical exam every six months. Keeping on top of these assessments was indirectly tied to reimbursement, since failure to comply would result in losing the organization's status for enhanced payments as a federal demonstration project. This threat was not abstract. After a biannual Centers for Medicare and Medicaid Services survey in April of 2011, the Grove had its license downgraded to provisional status. Although there were several documented deficiencies, the Grove's failure to meet assessment deadlines and to properly document those assessments became the primary focus of administrative interventions. The NPs were pressured to do the kind of work that counted on paper: medical work, not nursing work.

The clinicians at the Grove also had to keep in mind the preferences of their patients. While the Grove had a limited number of acceptable reasons to remove someone from its rolls, members had the unlimited right to leave the Grove and join a different Medicare- or Medicaid-funded program. If current members believed they were receiving something other than quality medical care, they might disenroll. The state collected data on the reasons for member disenrollment. The Grove was only one among many models that state and federal funders were considering. High levels of disenrollment due to program dissatisfaction would not bode well for its future.

But the need for competent care was not just a matter of customer satisfaction; the Grove's patient population had a high level of medical need. As NP Francesca observed, "The acuity level here is ridiculously high." Members and their families came to the clinic not just with complaints about transportation but with a long list of bodily complaints. They arrived with manageable, chronic conditions such as hypertension and diabetes. But they also arrived with less manageable chronic conditions such as renal failure, congestive heart failure, and multiple sclerosis. Moreover, they remained susceptible to acute conditions such as pneumonia, shingles, and urinary tract infections.

Whatever else the NPs chose to do, both payers and members expected them to address traditional medical problems as their core activity. To do so, they drew from the same well of interventions as physicians. In my fieldwork at Stanton School of Nursing, I observed that NP students were trained to rely on the evidence. While nursing's attention to whole person care was a core part of the curriculum, this professional axiom did not extend to substituting alternative practices for evidence-based approaches. Published guidelines for treatment decisions took center stage in the nursing classroom; these same guidelines were at the core of NP practice at the Grove. The work of the NPs was not separate from medical work, yet, their approach made it different from medical work. This modification of the medical counter inevitably raised questions about the work of the physicians.

Clinic Work as Nursing Difference

Managing the care of members as a team could not be done by email alone. Each team met weekly: Michelle's team on Wednesdays, Anne's team on Thursdays, and Norah's team on Fridays. Everyone on the core team was expected to attend: NPs, primary care nurses, physicians, physical therapists (PTs), occupational therapists (OTs), and social workers. The primary purpose of these meetings was twofold. First, the Grove was federally mandated to provide and document comprehensive assessments of members every six months. The primary work of the meeting was for each discipline to share its findings and make any adjustments to the member's plan of care. The other purpose of the meeting was to discuss "member issues." This was a residual category that contained a number of diverse problems. It might be a member request for additional home care hours, a complaint from transportation that a member was chronically late, or any problem that any staff member wanted the team to address.

Every team meeting would begin with the six-month assessments. Each clinician was asked to report on each member's status from his or her disciplinary perspective. Because this was the moment when everyone spoke from a specific arena of expertise, it was the part of the meeting where I had expected to see the most discussion, negotiation, and, perhaps, conflict. This expectation was almost never met. In some ways, this part of the meeting echoed the reading of lists during morning meeting. Everyone listened respectfully as the PT, social worker, and OT summarized their findings. The notes from the medical exam—sometimes performed by a physician, sometimes by an NP—were also quickly summarized. In some teams, the written notes from the medical exam were simply read aloud, often at a galloping pace that left no room for interruptions or conversation. In cases where the physician presented the assessment, the NPs might ask about a point of fact, but they neither questioned the assessment nor made suggestions. When NPs presented, a physician did sometimes make a recommendation. On these occasions, there would begin a carefully choreographed dance of civility. The physician would practice restraint, phrasing a recommendation as a suggestion rather than an order. "You may want to think about trying a different regimen for her hypertension," or "I've heard that Paxil is good for uremic itching. It's worth a try." The NPs replied with a practically jovial deference, with responses such as, "Oh, that's a good idea," or even more explicitly, "See, that's why you [the physician] are here."

The direct conflict over medical decision-making that I anticipated seeing was almost entirely absent. Within this organization, nurse managed though it was, physicians seemed to have uncontested authority over decisions that everyone recognized as being wholly medical. This state of affairs was not without some dissension. When I spoke with Francesca, she noted, "We have twenty-five people on the team; twenty-four agree and the physician says no and we still tend to go with the physician. So we've gotten into that authoritative kind of thing." For Francesca, this was part of a larger critique about the ways in which the Grove failed to live up to its nurse-managed ideals. And, in many ways, her observations matched my own. When a member problem was structurally demarcated as distinctly medical, the NPs' deference to physician authority was absolute.

However, in team meetings, these clinical assessments seemed only the pro forma prelude to what the meetings were really about: member issues. During this second part of the meeting, the team would debate and discuss such concerns as what to do about a member's cockroach problem that prevented home health care aides from providing regular care, or how to convince a member who was blind and had limited feeling in his extremities that he should consider moving into a supported living situation. These problems were rarely discrete or simple; consequently, conversations about them were long and prone to narrative exposition. Some team clinicians grumbled about the length and circuitousness of these discussions. Nonetheless, there was a high degree of participation, both through talking and through a posture of engaged listening from almost everyone present.

This was also the part of the meeting where NP knowledge was on full display. In team meetings, the NPs were the key weavers of member narratives. They shared information about their conversations with Mr. Whitmore's niece.

They recounted information about how Mr. Stiles's apartment used to look before his girlfriend moved in. They spoke about how Ms. Neville "was a success story" in terms of how difficult it had been to finally get her blood sugar under control. The NPs did not just share stories; they solicited them. Just as they opened the exam room to information that is usually filtered out of traditional medical encounters, they opened team meetings to the kind of storytelling that did not fit into the genre of case reports. The NPs displayed and added to their knowledge of members through team meetings. Yet in the context of sharing information, decisions *were* made. These decisions were not usually about medications or procedures, but from the NPs' perspective, they were important to the management of member care. Yet there seemed to be no explicitly medical decisions required.

The physicians, by their behavior, seemed to agree. During long conversations about member issues, the physicians normally multitasked by signing written orders or doing clinical work through smartphones. When opinions flew or stories were shared, the physicians' attention was usually elsewhere—if they were still at the meeting at all. Team meetings were usually rescheduled or cancelled altogether if an NP could not attend. Physician presence was treated as optional—by both the physicians and the team. When physicians' time was in short supply, they might arrive late, leave early, or skip the meeting entirely. In choosing to not participate in conversations that were not wholly medical, the physicians absented themselves from information sharing and decisions made about member care. In spite of NP deference to medical authority, physician authority was required for a shrinking proportion of member problems. As NP-defined clinic problems expanded, physician-defined medical problems seemed to contract.

Clinic Work as Expertise

The fact that the NPs had a deep level of knowledge about their members may have had an intangible value to members and their families. Perhaps this knowledge fostered a deeper sense of relationship between some members and some NPs. However, in the realm of medical care, such intangibles are rarely understood as goods in themselves. Indeed, we often tell stories about how the absence of such intangibles is in direct proportion to the more tangible rewards of better outcomes. For example, in the US, the iconic surgeon is someone whose technical skill is seen as so rarified that a lack of bedside manner is viewed almost as a consequence of that skill rather than a detriment to it. In comparison, bedside nurses may be idealized as being more nurturing than physicians, but their work is not thought to require much in the way of expertise. From this commonsense understanding of the world, it would not, then, be surprising to observe that NPs might have a more "nurturing" style of practice than physicians. We may be glad that nurses care, but we're not convinced it matters all that much for health outcomes.

This view of the world, however, has very little to do with the actual evidence, and a great deal more to do with gender. The historical division between medicine and nursing is grounded upon gendered notions of both skill and value: work done by women is seen as innate and therefore low skilled, while that done by men is seen as requiring expertise and is more highly valued. Yet nursing work is skilled work. Moreover, it requires a skill that study after study demonstrates is important not just for how patients "feel," but for whether patients thrive (Aiken 2014; Aiken et al. 2002; Blegen et al. 2013; Wong, Cummings, and Ducharme 2013). Similarly, the quantitative evidence suggests that the kind of care NPs provide is different not only in style from physicians but also in content and positive impact on patient health (Buerhaus et al. 2018; DesRoches et al. 2017; Martínez-González et al. 2014). My observations cannot speak to the impact of these NPs' clinical performance on patient outcomes, but they do show that this work was less about nurturing members than it was a distinctive approach to both seeing and solving problems. The knowledge NPs developed about members allowed them to cultivate a different form of expertise and to carry out a different form of work.

Anne had been an NP for over twenty years before coming to the Grove, but had spent most of that time in acute and institutional long-term care, rather than primary care. She remembered distinctly that when she arrived at the Grove, she had to hone not only her skills of diagnosis and treatment but also her approach to patient care.

> I mean, the first month I'm [at the Grove] and I get a lab result back; the PTINR [a measure of the rate of blood clotting] was high. So we needed to adjust the Coumadin dose. So you have to remember my background. My most recent places are working in a hospital, right? So I throw the order in the computer, I send it through to the nurse upstairs, I don't think twice about it. I get the next PTINR and it's still high. What happened? I forgot to call the family. You've got to do that in primary care. Transitioning into primary care from a lifetime of being in long-term care and acute care? It sucked. It sucked. There were just stumbling blocks everywhere.

When I met her, Anne was finishing her third year at the Grove. From my observations, she had clearly taken to heart the need to incorporate the family. One Wednesday, I spent a day shadowing her. As we approached late afternoon,

Anne was taking a moment of quiet to catch up on her email and write up notes for the electronic medical record. As was often the case, this small reprieve was interrupted by the ringing of the telephone. The caller was Susie, the oldest daughter of Ms. Gray. Susie described her mother as behaving nervously. Anne reported to Susie that she had seen Ms. Gray last week with a blood sugar level of four hundred. Ms. Gray had reportedly stopped taking her oral diabetes medication. Anne wondered aloud whether this sudden shift in behavior could be attributed to her diabetes and asked, "What's her blood sugar?" Susie didn't know but suggested that Anne call her younger sister, Tanisha. Susie had been tasked with calling Anne, but Tanisha was the daughter currently with Ms. Gray. Anne agreed, hung up, and called Tanisha. From the moment the line connected, Anne could hear why Ms. Gray's behavior change had seemed so urgent. While Anne was trying to speak with Tanisha, Ms. Gray was shouting so loudly in the background that it was difficult to carry on a conversation. Although we could not hear Ms. Gray's words, the anger behind them was unmistakable.

In spite of the chaos happening in the background, Anne began to troubleshoot what might be going on in order to piece together a plan of action. Ms. Gray had just returned home from a short hospital stay. Her routine prior to hospitalization was that when she did not attend the Grove's center, a nurse would make a home visit and administer her insulin injections. After some back and forth with Tanisha, Anne figured out that these nursing visits were never restarted after Ms. Gray returned home from her recent hospitalization. For most populations, insulin is self-administered. However, many older adults struggle to do so because of cognitive decline, fading memory, or just the difficulty of learning a new skill in later life. Although Ms. Gray had the support of two daughters, she lived by herself. Having assistance with insulin was one of the key supports that allowed her to live in her own home. Missing a few doses of insulin might not have been the entirety of the problem, but it was a good place to start. Anne ended the call by asking the daughter to try to check her mother's blood sugar and to call back with the result. While waiting for this new information, Anne did not return to her email or charting; she continued with the case of Ms. Gray. First, she sent off an email to the Grove's home care department. The email was only the first in a multistep process of both finding out why the nursing visits were not restarted and attending to the problem at hand by arranging for a nurse to make a home visit before the end of the day.

Anne's response to Ms. Gray's problem was an example of how the NPs' expansive notion of the clinical encounter involved taking members' and families' own constructions of the problem seriously. Ms. Gray's daughter had called as much out of frustration over her mother's rain of invectives as from a cool observation of changed behavior. Anne's openness to responding to this frustration was not only useful for short-term problem-solving. It was also part of how Anne was able to set the stage for longer-term management. To solve the problem, she reacquainted herself with both the medical record and the practicalities of Ms. Gray's care routines. Her approach to a clinical problem was to immerse herself in Ms. Gray's life, a life that included both domestic and organizational routines and relationships. In the context of troubleshooting a sudden behavior change, Anne found herself inside longstanding family dynamics and learning just a little more about each daughter's relationship to her mother. She also found herself solving the communication problems between the clinic and the home care department. Anne's openness to unfiltered complaints from members and their families was not just a reflection of an NP's orientation to patient care, but was constitutive of the NP's expertise. It was through this openness to information that the NPs became the resident experts of the Grove's members. And it was through that openness that they were able to marshal personal, family, and organizational resources to address member concerns.

The Grove's NPs had no interest in supplanting the expertise of the physicians. When faced with distinctly medical problems, the NPs used a variety of resources to make sure that they treated the concerns in the same ways a physician might. However, what I observed was that the NPs often faced different problems from those of their physician colleagues, not because they were leaving medical problems to the physicians, but because medical problems were often reconfigured as clinic problems.

In order to cultivate the expertise necessary to address these problems, the NPs paid attention to information from a range of sources. This attention was not passive but required an active stance of openness to both member and staff concerns. Through this openness, the NPs encountered clinical bodies that were embedded in social and organizational contexts. These bodies suffered from biological conditions as well as the exigencies of everyday life. And it was these bodies, rather than disease states, to which the NPs attended.

Clinic work made up the core of NP practice; it was also at the heart of the Grove's mission of coordinated care. Among elder care professionals, there is a saying: "The best long-term care insurance is a daughter." Even with Medicare and Medicaid paying for services, navigating bureaucracies and coordinating services is someone's full-time job. To categorize this as the work of daughters reveals it as the kind of invisible work that money does not easily buy. For many, these idealized daughters are in short supply. Few families have access to a physically healthy adult whose time is not taken up by work in the paid labor market or by unpaid responsibilities such as caring for dependent children. Moreover, the work of coordination is not unskilled labor; an adult's availability does not necessarily signal possession of the knowledge or skill to do what needs to be done.

For many of its members, the Grove had become an organizational daughter. Yet how good a daughter it proved to be seemed to depend largely on the work of the NP. To the extent that coordination happened at all, it happened through NP expertise. This observation is not to diminish the work of anyone else on the team. I went on home visits with the OTs, watched the PTs work with members in the gym, and sat in the offices of the social workers. Everyone did their part, and everyone cared for members. However, the work of navigating hurdles and coordinating care was carried out primarily by the NPs from inside the clinic. It was their knowledge of members lives *and* of the organizational context that positioned them as the providers who knew how to solve the problems that inevitably arise when delivering so many different forms of care. The NPs remained responsible for the treatment of member complaints. Whether these complaints were a product of biological, social, or organizational ills, the NPs expanded the medical encounter to include them. Their performance of clinic work was not simply an addition to medical work; it was a transformation of it.

The transformative quality of clinic work puts it in conversation with the well-studied concept of medicalization. Medicalization describes the processes through which problems not previously amenable to medical work come to be seen as such (Conrad 1992, 2007). The transformation of grief into depression and of childhood unruliness into attention deficit disorder are both examples of medicalization. To offer these examples is not necessarily to put forward a critique. For many, medicalization eases suffering, either through access to effective treatments or simply by making suffering comprehensible. However, medicalization has consequences beyond the scope of the individual patient. To define a condition as a medical concern removes it from other realms of authority. When grief becomes depression, it is no longer at home in the church or synagogue, but is now most appropriately addressed in the offices of psychiatrists. Medicalization not only changes the arsenal of solutions at our disposal; it also changes what we consider our problems to be (Freidson 1988b; Hughes 1981).

I invoke medicalization more as sensitizing concept (Blumer 1954) than as precise description. Since the original explication of medicalization, it has been updated and amended with the observation that the process involves not only physicians but also pharmaceutical companies, lawyers, payers, and patients. Despite this ever-expanding list of the "engines" of medicalization (Conrad 2005), nursing has never been theorized as one. Nursing possesses neither the generative power to create new conditions nor the constraining power to hold medicine's domain in check. Indeed, my descriptions of clinic work illustrate that expansions of nursing authority in the medical encounter are seemingly matched by the increasing power of patients and the health care organization. However, a focus on what nursing is not doing within realms of knowledge obscures the work it is doing inside organizations.

At the Grove, clinic work transformed local, organizational understandings of what kinds of problems counted as medical problems. Members and families who turned to the clinic with a broad set of concerns had them met. The responses of the NPs reshaped their expectations about what kinds of problem could be solved in the medical encounter. Staff too brought problems to the clinic, changing the encounter from one solely between patient and provider to one that included the organization. Although the NPs did not offer new diagnoses or treatments, their responsiveness eased the suffering of their patients nonetheless. In widening the clinic's doors to new kinds of problems, the NPs were quite effective at expanding everyday understandings of what was amenable to nursing expertise, as well as what could be addressed in the medical encounter.

ORGANIZATIONAL CARE WORK

In their performance of clinic work, the NPs encountered all manner of member problems, whether they were brought by the members themselves, by family, or by staff. Solving these problems involved both clinical knowledge and the work of weaving together both family and organizational resources. However, clinic work was not limited to addressing member problems; it often meant dealing with those faced by the organization. "The Grove," NP Norah was fond of saying, "is like a funnel. Everything rolls down to the nurse practitioner." For Norah, this image was an evocation of the centrality of her work; the NP was uniquely poised to be the connector and chief narrator of member needs. Norah's analogy had been taken up by others, but with a slightly different emphasis.

When NP Michelle repeated Norah's analogy, she began by saying, "At the Grove, all the problems come in like a big funnel. They go all the way down to the nurse practitioner to solve." To make sure I understood, she elaborated: "The NPs have to do everything. . . . We're in charge of remembering everything." For Michelle, the NPs were not choosing to solve a broad range of problems out of professional mission; they were doing so out of obligation. Certainly, the needs of members were part of this obligation, but for Michelle, the pressure to stand at the bottom of an organizational funnel came directly from her employer.

In this chapter, I look more closely at the ways in which the NPs' performance of clinic work was at once a professional responsibility and an organizational one. Although the Grove's model pressed all its providers toward more diffuse definitions of work, the responsibility to resolve distinctly organizational problems was unique to the NPs. In particular, the pressure to do so from inside the clinic was not felt by the physicians. Despite an organizational logic of interchangeability, clinic work was not medical work, and the physicians were not NPs. The enacted distinctions between NP and physician work were not the result of an agreed-upon division of labor. Rather, they were a function of who had the power to say no to organizational concerns. At the same time, the NPs' obligations to dispatch what I call organizational care work did not absolve them from attending to medical concerns. Instead they were asked to carry out the mission of the organization as an integral part of what it meant to medically care for members. The NPs were not just doing different work from the physicians; they were doing so as very different kinds of organizational actors. The NPs' performance of organizational care work was crucial to how the Grove fulfilled its mission of comprehensive care; however, like other forms of care work, it was neither always visible nor recognized as requiring expertise.

The Problem with the NPs

"Why are the NPs emailing transportation?" For NP Stephen, the Grove's director of nursing, this was a rhetorical question. He was not interested in solving a problem of transportation; he was interested in solving his problem with the NPs. Like most health care organizations, the Grove maintained separate chains of command for nurses and physicians. Although the NPs and physicians were both hired to attend to medical needs, the Grove had a physician as medical director and an NP as its director of nursing. Stephen had only been on the job for a few months, but it did not take him long to raise questions about what he saw the NPs doing. He had attended scores of morning meetings and witnessed the NPs' broad set of preoccupations. He was also, like every administrator, on each team's email list. He read the never-ending stream of emails about medications, coordination problems, and transportation woes. Stephen felt he had a clear view of how the NPs spent their time. So when he asked why the NPs were emailing transportation, he was alluding to a well-substantiated critique about their work: the NPs were busy doing things they should not be doing.

Stephen may have been a newcomer to the Grove, but he was not new to nursing. He had worked as an RN for almost a decade before he became educated and licensed as an NP. As an insider, he was well versed with the uncertainty that was endemic to the NPs' role. "The NPs' role," he explained, "is still under construction, as I'm sure you've observed. Because depending on the state in which you're practicing, you either have a narrow[er] or a wider scope [of practice]." This uncertainty was not just a reflection of regulations; it was embedded in workplace logics. Stephen described having fought a three-year battle with administration over NP work in his previous job. "They saw the NPs as 'super RNs' and wanted to use them as RNs. They just did not understand the role." Despite his personal experience with the external pressures on NPs, as an administrator at the Grove, he had a concrete, internal problem he needed to address. "The NPs," he told me, "have to unlearn being RNs."

Stephen was not the only administrator who had a problem with the NPs. Dr. Christine Morgan, the Grove's medical director, was often perplexed by what she saw the NPs doing. For her, the natural comparison for the NPs was not other nurses, but physicians. "Physicians are very protective of our time; very protective. . . . I mean, I know [the members] need to ask something. But I know if I stop and take that question, not only will I be enrolled in whatever they ask, but there are four other people sitting there who will want to do the same thing. But the NPs don't protect their time."

When Christine first arrived at the Grove, she could not understand this behavior. She had never worked closely with NPs before, but if their purpose was to do the work of physicians, there was no reason for them to act so differently. Stephen's hiring helped to supply an answer. When he arrived, the two of them began talking with one another as well as working together. As administrators, their offices were on the third floor—an elevator ride away from the clinic, but only steps from one another. They shared information about the practical aspects of organizing the clinical work at the Grove and had conversations bordering on the philosophical about the relationship between nursing and medicine. From these frequent talks with Stephen, Christine had developed an explanation about the NPs' behavior as rooted in nursing's responsiveness as a profession. As Christine talked to me about what the NPs did in the clinic, she noted, "Stephen told me it was a nursing thing . . . this idea of 'bring it on; I'll do it.'" This analysis, however, made her neither appreciative nor particularly sympathetic. "The [NPs' list] of other duties keeps getting longer and longer. And it's not getting longer and longer because somebody 'up here' is telling them it needs to get longer and longer. It's getting longer and longer because they're just like, 'I'll do it. Bring it on. I'll do it.'. . . They're doing all this other stuff that they don't need to."

For Christine, the NPs' insistence on doing "stuff that they don't need to" was not just a waste of time; it was a dereliction of duty. It got in the way of practicing medicine. Christine was one of several people at the Grove with whom I shared my analysis of clinic work. In one of our recorded interviews, I can be heard describing the NPs as "spiderweb people" who seem to be everywhere at once. "I mean," I said, "they sit in the clinic, but they are everywhere. They are in the members' homes, their bedrooms, and inside transportation. Through the phone and email, they are in all of these places and doing all of these things all day long. For them, this has become medical management." At this last statement, Christine halted my overly admiring description by interjecting: "But it's not! That's not medical management!"

As well as rejecting the NPs' embodiment of medical management, Christine struggled to see it as a valid form of expertise. She was not, for example, enamored with the NPs' practice of acting as the conduit of member needs. While I was doing my fieldwork, nursing homes were reluctant to use NPs to meet the regulatory requirement of having a medical provider see residents every six months. The NPs could be the provider of record at the Grove, but when members entered the nursing home, whether for rehab or long-term care, the physicians had to fill this role. However, when nursing home staff had a question or need concerning a member, it was often easier to call the usually answered NP number rather than to chance being routed to the physician's voice mail. The NPs, acting as air traffic controllers, would invariably take the call and either solve the problem directly or relay the message to the responsible physician. Either way, the nursing home staff had spoken with a person and their responsibility had been discharged.

This behavior by the NPs frustrated Christine. "Why are you now becoming my secretary? A physician would *never* do that." Christine wanted the NPs to respond to these phone calls in the same way a physician would. "'You don't need to talk to me.' *Click.* 'Why are you calling me? This is not something I need to be involved in. You need to speak to so and so. Goodbye. End of conversation.' ... I mean, can I do that? Sure! I can take a message with the best of them. I was a secretary for my dad when I was sixteen. I know all about taking messages. But am I going to? Not in this lifetime." For Christine, the NPs' insistence on "taking messages" was not what it meant to practice medicine. She had learned early on that "you have to say no. You have to train yourself to say no." Both Stephen and Christine agreed that the behavior of the NPs needed to change. For Stephen, the NPs needed to stop acting like RNs. For Christine, they needed to start behaving more like physicians.

There are many NPs who would disagree with Christine's assessment. In the time I spent among NPs in training at Stanton, I found that students and faculty circulated narratives that asserted that NP skill would not come from striving to be "like doctors" but from "remembering to be nurses." Nursing has given NPs a way of understanding their role as different from just doing what a physician might (Trotter 2019). From their perspective, it is not necessarily a problem that physicians might not always recognize the work of the NP as being identical to their own. But there was at least one NP who might have agreed with Christine.

For Michelle, the work at the Grove was a challenge. In most ways, it was one she relished. Although she had been an NP for over twenty years, the Grove was her first job in outpatient care. When she took the position, she knew there would be a learning curve. Michelle explained, "I had never really done this kind of nurse practitioner work where you're really in charge." But she was up for the clinical challenge, noting, "I wanted to see if I could do it." However, there were other challenges at the Grove about which she was less enthusiastic.

For Michelle, the feeling of having to "do everything" was not just an annoyance; it was a burden. She experienced the never-ending cascade of emails, phone calls, and staff visitations as "constant interruptions." She described having to make her own clinic schedule and put in her own lab orders as examples of the larger NP obligation "to remember everything." The expectation of needing to respond to all these needs made her feel as if "[the NPs] aren't in charge. Everyone else is." The Grove may have been nurse-managed, but Michelle didn't see much evidence that the NPs "ran anything." She laughed as she said, "Nurse-run? It runs on the backs of the NPs!"

Michelle's words were not just free-standing grumblings; they were born from a direct comparison with an ideal of how the Grove might have been organized. What Michelle really wanted was for the Grove to run "more like a doctor's office." She did not necessarily mind being the coordinator of member care. I listened to her say on more than one occasion to a member's son or daughter, "Give me a call if there is a problem; I'm the point person." However, she would rather have had someone else address problems with van drivers, home care aides, and missed appointments. Michelle wanted to be responsible for medical care rather than caught at the end of an organizational funnel. Her critique and comparative ideal matched those of Stephen and Christine in every way but one: Michelle did not believe she did this work out of a nurse's commitment to "bring it on; I'll do it." She did it because she believed it was what her employer required her to do. Perhaps Michelle, like Christine, could have trained herself to say no. There were, however, consequences to saying no. Before addressing these, I will first consider why the NPs so often said yes.

On the Backs of the NPs

When Christine implied that the NPs would be better clinicians if they behaved more like physicians, she was invoking the logic of interchangeability. Using this logic, the more closely NP practices match those of physicians, the better. Although the Grove was a nurse-managed organization, it too had an explicit logic of NP and physician interchangeability. From the organization's perspective, either an NP or a physician could solve the kinds of problems that members brought to the clinic. There were times, however, when the validity of this logic was tested. One of those moments was when an NP went on vacation.

In March of 2011, it was announced in morning meeting that Norah would be away from the clinic for almost two weeks. As part of that announcement, staff were advised to refer all member issues to Dr. Tracy Polson. At the beginning of my fieldwork, there had been a number of staff separations and new people hired. At the physician level, there had been an almost complete turnover. In addition to a new medical director, Tracy was one of two full-time physicians who had been hired to supplement the one part-time physician who remained. This was potentially a new chapter for the Grove. In one of our interviews, Stephen pointed out that "historically, the Grove had never had full-time physicians. They were all part-time. We never even had a full-time medical director. . . . So what does it mean, in a nurse-managed place like this is, to have three-and-a-half physicians?"

The fact that the full-time physicians were relatively new hires brought an additional level of uncertainty around how they might work with the NPs. It was not just a question of how physicians and NPs should work together, but of how *these* physicians and *these* NPs would do so. By the time of Norah's vacation, the Grove had settled into a configuration whereby an NP anchored each team, and the physicians were shared across two teams. This arrangement seemed to strike a solid balance between the ideal of NP leadership with the one of teamwork. This was the balance at work when administration announced that while Norah was out, concerns about her members should be forwarded to Tracy. Since both NPs and physicians were medically responsible for their teams, it made sense that one could be asked to fill in for the other. However, as I listened to this announcement, I began to wonder how this directive would take shape in a context in which clinic work had largely subsumed medical work. Would Tracy's phone begin ringing nonstop? Would receptionists and clerks start lining up outside her door? Would she begin answering emails addressed to the team about issues with transportation and medication delivery? None of these things occurred. What I observed was that when physicians were asked to fill in for NPs, they mostly did not.

Announcements from administration aside, when the NPs were out, staff did not relay member concerns to a physician. They relayed these concerns to the primary care nurse. In part, this was a function of the responsiveness of these nurses. When Norah was in the clinic, RN Joanne had her own work to do. She had state-mandated nursing assessments to complete that were separate from the medical assessments. She had members whom she followed on her own, such as Mr. Stout, whom she called every day to remind to take his insulin. But in other ways, she and Norah worked as a team. Much of what Norah knew about her members, she shared with Joanne. Their offices faced each other, which made Joanne the perfect audience for Norah's habit of announcing everything that happened during the day.

As a result of these exchanges, Joanne had a great deal of member knowledge to marshal in Norah's absence. Joanne used that knowledge to attend to many of the phone calls, hallway visits, and doorway consultations to which Norah might have attended. Although no one had announced the new burdens on the primary care nurse that Norah's absence would cause, Joanne already knew what to expect. On Norah's first day of vacation, I asked Joanne whether I could follow her. "I want to see what your day is like when Norah is out." Joanne firmed her lips and said quietly, "babysitting." At the time I thought she meant babysitting the members with their unending complaints. Then I began to wonder whether she meant she would be babysitting the physicians. But by the end of the first week, it seemed to me that her description was not about any one person's work or set of tasks. In Norah's absence, Joanne seemed to be babysitting the organization as she took on the extra burdens of clinic work.

In some ways, the ability of Joanne to take on some of Norah's work was compatible with Stephen's analysis. There were aspects of what the NPs did that could be done by a capable RN. This observation, however, is not unique to the Grove. Ethnographic accounts of hospital work are full of illustrations of how seemingly solid boundaries between professions are crossed and blurred in the everyday welter of getting the job done (Allen 2001; Apesoa-Varano 2013; Apesoa-Varano and Varano 2014; Evers 1982; Roth and Douglas 1983; Sudnow 1967; Zerubavel 1979). Medical residents learn fairly quickly that if floor nurses do not make some independent "medical" decisions, their own workload goes from challenging to untenable (Kellogg 2011; Allen 1997).

In my observations, Joanne stepped, quite nimbly, into the breach of Norah's absence. But she did not do so purely from a professional stance of "bring it on; I'll do it." Joanne did not actively seek out these new problems to solve; they were systematically brought to her door. Member calls that normally went to Norah were rerouted to the clinic receptionist. The receptionist chose to forward these calls to Joanne, not the physician. So when the dialysis center had a concern about a member's condition, it was Joanne who received the call. When the medical assistants taking routine vitals found an elevated blood pressure, it was not the physician they sought out; it was Joanne. In a notable example, one of the receptionists came back to the clinic with a message from a member's wife. She stopped first at Michelle's door. Upon hearing the name of the member, Michelle declared, "Oh, he's not on my team. I think he belongs to Norah." The staff member then walked right past Tracy's open door—the physician who was ostensibly filling in for Norah—made her way down the hall, and delivered the message to Joanne.

For many member needs, Joanne proved herself perfectly capable of acting as the air traffic controller. But there were some parts of Norah's job that Joanne had to refer to someone else. On the fourth day of Norah's vacation, one of her members was discharged from the hospital. When members were released from the hospital to home, there was a standard organizational protocol that required them to be brought to the Grove's clinic before being taken home. During that clinic visit, the NP would address unanswered questions about any hospital interventions that might have been done, make a note of any needed follow-up, and assess and update the plan of care. In Norah's absence, the member was automatically added to the physician's schedule. Tracy would be expected to do what Norah would have normally done. This is not what happened.

Part of Tracy's role outside the clinic was to manage members in the hospital. Earlier that morning, she had completed rounds at the hospital and had been the physician who had officially discharged the member. On seeing the familiar name on her roster, she told Joanne, "I already saw her. She's fine to go home. I don't need to see her again." Joanne tried to explain that there were things that had to be done after discharge. But after making no headway with her requests, Joanne eventually found someone who would do the work that needed to be done: NP Alice, a part-time NP from another team. Although Tracy had not seen any medical work that needed to be done, Alice discovered that there was plenty of clinic work to do.

I watched as Alice spent the next thirty-five minutes making phone calls, sending emails, updating the chart, and faxing in prescriptions. There were changes to the member's medication that had to be explained as well as internally ordered. There were changes that needed to happen at home. As is often the case, the member was going home at a lower level of physical functioning than before and needed an order for additional hours with a home care aide. There were family caregivers to call. She needed to make sure they understood what had changed and how they might need to adjust their own level of support. She had to read through the discharge paperwork, compare it with the member's status before hospitalization, and make a note about what needed to be updated in the member's plan of care. Because she was a part-time NP, this was not exactly routine work for Alice. Yet it was not entirely unfamiliar. It was not all that different from what she did for members every day, which she described as taking responsibility for the "big picture" that helped her keep members "functional." Part-time or full-time, exemplary or less so, this was the work of every NP at the Grove. It was not, however, the work of the physicians.

As a physician, Tracy undoubtedly had her own sense of professional responsibility. Moreover, she was a geriatrician, a primary care specialty that has its own holistic point of view. It was Norah who explained to me that geriatricians "can't help but look at a patient as a system rather than just one disease process or one elderly lady." But in spite of this potential concordance between the ideological holism of NPs and geriatricians, Tracy could not see her own work reflected in that of the NPs. It was clear that what clinic protocol required from Tracy in the NP's absence was not just work that she was unaccustomed to doing, but work that she did not know was being done. Tracy neither did the work herself nor delegated it to someone else. She knew that the Grove coordinated care, but she did not really understand the work required to make that happen, let alone who did it.

In contrast, coordinating care was the standard work of all the Grove's NPs. Alice was not even a full-time NP, yet her actions indicated that she knew more about how the Grove's organizational structure functioned than a full-time physician. This was not because Alice had keener powers of observation, nor was it because she affectively cared more for the members. It was because knowing this structure was a required part of her job. In the absence of formal divisions of labor, organizational charts, or job descriptions, the NPs had developed a way of doing the job of which even the administrators who ran the organization did not seem fully aware. The physicians could not fill in for NPs because they did not know what the job entailed, nor did they have the requisite knowledge about members or the organization to carry it out.

It was also clear that this work was not just for the benefit of members; it was at the heart of the Grove's organizational promise. The Grove needed the NPs to say yes to this work in order to carry out its own mission of coordinated care. The obligation of the NPs to say yes cannot be viewed apart from the physicians' lack of obligation to do the same. In Norah's absence, the physician was asked to do the work of coordination. The physician, however, declined. Moreover, it was not just this NP's vacation, or this team, or this physician. The NPs had made repeated observations of physician refusal. One NP recounted that when a physician was previously asked to cover for a missing NP colleague, "I had her nurse in and out of my office all day. I had her appointment clerk in and out of my office. And [another NP] did two of her enrollments. What exactly," she asked rhetorically, "did the physician do?"

The physicians' pattern of declining to do clinic work was a reality not only for the NPs but also for other staff. During Norah's vacation, I observed that staff routinely turned to Joanne to solve team problems. There was a reason why phone calls and messages and hallway consultations were routed to someone other than the physician. The primary care nurses were not the only ones to face physician refusal. Other staff members described the physicians as "less approachable" than the NPs. There was the appointment clerk who found the physicians lacking when compared to the NPs who, if she needed something, "it's done." There was the staff member who shared that "[the physicians] make me not want to engage . . . they can sometimes be kind of bullying in that they dictate to you what they want." Another staff member described bringing a member problem, which the worker felt had a medical component, to a physician and being chastised with an exasperated "Can't you solve this problem on your own?" Although I only had access to one side of this story, the key aspect of the narrative was less the alleged impatience of the physician and more the moral taken from it: "If I had brought the problem to [my team's NP], she would have never yelled at me like that."

Whether physician refusal in any one instance was from lack of knowledge or from unwillingness, the practical result was the same. The Grove's staff had learned that member problems should be directed to a nurse—an NP if available, but another nurse if not—and not a physician. The NPs had become a resource that anyone could deploy. The NPs' professional openness was an invitation for anyone in the organization to bring problems that they could not solve to the clinic. By contrast, the physicians resisted being deployed by anyone other than themselves. No one disputed their clinical abilities or the quality of care they provided. The physicians had the organization's respect, but no one saw them as an organizational resource.

Organizational Obligations

To be a resource, of course, is one thing. To have the organization run on your back is quite another. These two sides of the same reality were reflected not only in how the NPs experienced their work but also in how the organization evaluated them. There was a broad if informal consensus that Norah was one of the best NPs. While some believed this evaluation reflected her clinical acumen, there was no organizational data I could find that made this more than a subjective truth. However, subjective truths are not always without foundation. Certainly, Norah was one of the more confident NPs. I also found her to be somewhat charismatic. Her organizational presentation of self was as solid as anything else I observed about her. This mix of confidence and charisma might have shaped how her colleagues viewed her as well as how members experienced her bedside manner.

However, Norah's presentation of self was not the only thing that was different about her. Of all the NPs I observed in practice, she was the most adept at carrying the responsibility to do everything, remember everything, and act as the frontline fixer of a range of organizational problems. As I followed her, I watched her stabilize uncontrolled hypertension, figure out why this member or that refused to get on the van, and get to the bottom of discrepancies between what aides observed and what families reported. All the NPs performed an expansive notion of clinic work, but Norah was the exemplar. She was the NP who was most likely to say yes. But more importantly, after saying yes, she was the NP most likely to deliver on that promise. A core part of her skill was in how she addressed problems before they arose. The work involved in making this happen was easier to see when things did not go as planned.

There were days when I followed the NPs as a literal shadow. There were other days when I observed from a vantage point that provided a wider view of the action. Norah's habit of yelling things across the hall to Joanne made the spot outside her door an attractive place to stand. On one of these days, I stood outside her door and listened as she received a phone call. It was from Sheila, and she was not happy. "My mom did not see the dentist today. Why not?" It was a simple question, but also a complex one. Ms. Millie, Sheila's mother, had been on the list to see the dentist who visited the Grove once a month. Being on this list itself required some specific acts of coordination. If the dentist was scheduled for a Tuesday, members who did not normally attend on that day had to come in on a day outside their normal routines. Van drivers had to have their routes altered. The schedules of unpaid family caregivers, as well as paid aides who bathed, dressed, and fed members, might have to be adjusted. Many things could go wrong. But in the case of Ms. Millie, everything seemed to have gone right. She had been on the list. Transportation had brought her to the Grove on the right day. An aide had brought her back to the dentist that morning. So Norah was understandably perplexed when Sheila called. "She didn't? I swear I *saw* her physically get into the dentist's chair." Norah told Shelia to "hold on." She was going to figure it out. She put down the phone and walked across the hall to speak with the appointment clerk. As they talked, the fuller story unfolded. Ms. Millie had indeed gotten into the dentist's chair, but the dentist had instructed her to return after lunch. That is where the problem began.

Joanne explained to me, "It's hard. Because once the aides bring someone back, they cross them off their list. They're done. So then we have to remember to go find them if they themselves don't or won't remember to come back on their own." Many of the Grove's members had failing memories. Others required help to physically navigate the center. The organization had a routine for bringing Ms. Millie to the dentist the first time. But the dentist, working as an outside contractor, was not a part of this routine. She had, quite erroneously, treated Ms. Millie as the manager of her own schedule and entrusted her with the directive to return later. Consequently, Ms. Millie did not make it back onto any aide's list. And therefore, she did not see the dentist.

Norah explained the situation to the daughter and apologized, adding, "I will make sure she sees the dentist next time." But that afternoon was the first of many telephone conversations with Sheila. There was the time the dentist's visit coincided with a day Norah was out; she had not been there to make sure the visit happened. There was the time when the blood thinner Ms. Millie was on needed to be stopped prior to a dental procedure, but the medication nurse who filled her medi-set, a prefilled weekly pillbox, had not gotten the message to remove the pill in time. The problem with Ms. Millie was not a simple one, but Norah found herself on the front lines of making sure it got solved. This reality helped to explain why the NPs went over all their member's appointments, including internal appointments such as seeing the dentist. On a different day, I watched Norah go over the dentist list that the clerk had emailed. Norah, being Norah, sat at her desk and read the list aloud. "Mr. Reeves, yes. Ms. Blackmore, uh huh. Wait. Ms. Crawford should *not* be on there, but Delores Franklin should!" I watched Norah jump up from her chair and go across the hall to talk to the appointment clerk. "Ms. Franklin *has* to see the dentist. The family wants her to see the dentist." When the clerk asked why, Norah replied, "I don't know and I don't care. Her family wants her to see the dentist. She. Has. To. Be. Seen." After returning to her office, Norah turned to me and confided, "I wish I didn't have to be responsible for whether Ms. Franklin gets to see the dentist or not. It becomes my job to personally escort someone back to the dentist chair." She explained that she was the one "who gets screamed at" when members did not get what they needed. Just as Stephen had asked me, "Why are the NPs emailing transportation?" I might imagine him rhetorically asking, "Why are the NPs going over dentist appointments?" The answer to both is the same. When an NP faltered, clinic problems quickly became organizational problems.

NP Anne may not have been put forward as one of the best NPs, but she took her performance of clinic work seriously. She also knew that there were times when she faltered at the work of remembering everything. One morning, I watched Anne make her way through a small pile of papers on her desk. When I asked about the provenance of this pile, she responded that various people "drop all manner of papers in my inbox, put them on my desk, put them on my chair—anything that says my team." Some of these pieces of paper were lab results. Some were specialist consults. Some were notifications of follow-up appointments that an outside specialist's office had made instead of the Grove's appointment clerks. Each piece of paper represented what someone perceived as an NP responsibility.

Anne then proceeded to recount a cautionary tale of the time she took one day too many to get through her stack of papers. One of her members had been scheduled for a swallowing study. That piece of paper had been added to her pile earlier in the week; she came across it as she was trying to clear off her desk on a Friday evening. The appointment was for Monday at ten in the morning. Knowing all the work required to get members from one place to another, Anne did her best to make it happen. She sent an email to transportation with the request, as per protocol. Even as she clicked send, she knew it was a futile gesture. It was already six; the transportation staff had gone home. But Anne had an idea. She called the cell phone of her appointment clerk who, it turned out, was out having dinner with the transportation coordinator. They talked everything over. It seemed as though the appointment might happen after all. Everyone said it would work out. But it didn't.

Between the six-o'clock phone call and the end of the night, the transportation coordinator had forgotten to follow through. No one notified the member. No one arranged for her transportation. The swallowing study had to be rescheduled. Anne was sanguine. "It's understandable," she said. "These things happen." In hindsight, she reconsidered relying on someone's memory after they were officially off the clock and out on a Friday night. It was a mistake, but ultimately, it was Anne's mistake. If everyone could go back in time and "do things right," the solution would have been for Anne to have done something differently. She should have gone through the pile of papers faster. She should have paid closer attention to the needs of her members.

Anne found it difficult to prioritize getting through the stack of undifferentiated pieces of paper every day, and she recognized that this problem sometimes had consequences for members. "If it's a follow-up appointment that happens in a month? No problem. But if it's an appointment that happens in a week? That could be a problem." The NPs' attention to every detail of their members' care began to take on new meaning. It was a story that drove home the reality that the Grove's promise of care coordination seemed to depend upon the NPs' direct attention to every phone call, every email, and every piece of paper that made it to their desks. The NPs were not just taking on responsibility; they were often held responsible when things did not go smoothly.

At the Grove, Norah was an exemplary NP both because she said yes and because she was the most likely to successfully follow through. Other NPs said yes but were successful less often. There was another option. They could have said no. They might have declined to take on the responsibility for transportation, for getting members to appointments, for making sure families were really on board for postoperative care. Both the director of nursing and the medical director had put this forward as the best option—not only for the NPs but also for their members. From their vantage point outside the clinic, they believed that if the NPs could just bring themselves to say no, they'd have more time for the medical work that really mattered. However, just as there were accolades for "one of the best NPs" when she said yes, there were consequences for the NP who said no.

Michelle was the NP who most reliably said no. First, I will say that in many ways, Michelle did say yes to many aspects of clinic work. She said yes to the coordination work of helping members like Ms. Payne prepare for surgery. She said yes to the work of listening to members like Mr. George, who brought both emergent concerns with congestive heart failure and less urgent questions about medication side effects. Moreover, she was not exempt from the way the Grove structurally relied upon NP availability. All her members and their families had access to her direct office number. Michelle received her own set of complaints about specialist appointments, medication delivery, and transportation. After closely observing Michelle's day, however, I began to notice that she often made very different choices about how to respond.

Michelle was the last NP I shadowed. After spending only a couple of days with her, I was viscerally struck by one defining difference between her and the other NPs: her telephone was comparatively silent. In that first week, her daily average number of calls from members and their families was seven. By comparison, I counted an average of sixteen such telephone calls for Norah, which did not include the voice mails from the calls she did not take. Given that the majority of member calls were directly dialed rather than transferred from the front desk, the difference could not be explained by staff behavior; the reason had to lie with the members. Why did Michelle's members behave so differently?

My first observation was that although Michelle received calls, she did not cultivate them. If a family called about transportation, she would listen to their complaints, but she would end the call by giving them transportation's direct number. If a patient called about a problem with a missed specialist appointment, she would listen, but then she would tell them to call the appointment clerk. Because she did not take on the role of complaint conduit, Michelle's members never learned to call her first. This difference in responsiveness began even before the encounter. The other NPs checked voice mail and returned phone calls throughout the day. They behaved as if the phone was just as important as an in-person patient encounter. By contrast, Michelle would triage her calls; only urgent "sick" calls would be prioritized. When a member left a message about stomach pain, Michelle would return the call on the same day. Other calls might not be returned until the next day or the day after. By not performing responsiveness, Michelle effectively eliminated herself as the first line for member complaints.

She did the same for staff. When staff members brought complex problems to her doorway, she did not always, as Norah did, spring into action. At first, I was struck by how much she relied on the skills of other people on her team, from her clerk to her primary care nurse to the occupational therapist. She did this not only in the case of organizational problems such as transportation or appointments but also with clinical problems that could be addressed by other health care professionals. When action could be taken, she would sometimes respond, but she would just as often refer. She was, it seemed, doing exactly what Stephen and Christine believed the NPs should do. She could not change the way the clinic was organized, but she had learned to say no. In my naivete, I initially understood this as a positive quality. But that was before I began to see evidence that the Grove had a different understanding of Michelle's decisions. Michelle received no accolades for standing up and saying no. Instead, she became "the disorganized NP" on the "disorganized team."

One afternoon, I found myself in the third-floor hallway, having an impromptu conversation with a staff member in an administrative role. At one point, this person opined to me that Norah was the individual on her team who seemed to "know the whole case." This pronouncement was not made within a context of praising Norah, but to comparatively criticize Michelle. This person shared that Michelle's style was "disorganized." I first took this conversation lightly; to be noted, surely, but no different from dozens of off-the-cuff opinions I would hear about a coworker. Everyone had their favorite PT; everyone had their least favorite aide. But the content of this and other conversations about Michelle was more than idle gossip; it would ultimately manifest as its own organizational belief.

Almost six months after I had finished observing Michelle, I decided to drop in to her part of the clinic to say hello. But before I could get there, I heard the news from one of the primary care nurses. A few days before, Michelle had been told that "administration" was switching her primary care nurse with that of another team. The nurse fumed that administration had called Michelle's team disorganized—unfairly, in her estimation. I made my way down to Michelle's office and asked her directly: Did she know why they were changing her nurse? She repeated the same reason I had just heard—administration considered her team disorganized. I heard the same explanation from RN Claudia, Michelle's soon-to-be-former primary care nurse. There was something about how Michelle did her job that the Grove's administration found in need of intervention. But it was not, apparently, the work she was explicitly hired to do: provide medical care. It is entirely possible that Michelle's clinical skills were not as good as Norah's. I do not have the requisite data to make that assessment; neither, however, did the Grove. According to the NPs and the director of nursing, provider-specific information on patient outcomes was neither collected nor analyzed. Rather, it was Michelle's "disorganization" that triggered administrative action.

What disorganization meant was clear from the solution offered. After Michelle's team was diagnosed as disorganized, the specific intervention was not to modify the behavior of the physician, social worker, OT, or PT. Nor was it to provide team-wide training in skills of collaboration or delegation. Underscoring that the problem was not about clinical expertise, there was no suggestion that Michelle work more closely with her team's physician (or that the physician work more closely with her). The solution that the Grove put forward was to give Michelle's team a different nurse. What Michelle was failing at was not treated as medical work but as nursing work. Stephen may have thought the NPs needed to unlearn being RNs, but it seemed that Michelle's refusal to be an RN had become an organizational problem. Christine may have believed the NPs should behave more like physicians; however, when an NP attempted to protect her time like a physician, the result extended beyond hallway grumblings and manifested as formal administrative censure. The NP who refused to engage in organizational care work was not praised; she was reprimanded.

The NP as Organizational Actor

The Grove ran more smoothly when someone stepped in to solve the everyday problems of coordination. The NPs became that someone from a mixture of professional responsibility and organizational obligation. The depth of that obligation requires some explanation. While clients and consumers often prefer that organizations run more effectively, doing so is not always an organizational priority. Why the NPs' performance of organizational care work mattered to the Grove and not just to its members bears some consideration. The success or failure to coordinate care had consequences for members, but it also had consequences for the Grove's bottom line.

I did not spend much time with the Grove's members who had transitioned to permanent nursing home residence, but one such experience stayed with me. The Grove contracted with several nursing homes for its members, of which Ellington Court was one. Ellington was not one of the nicer nursing homes, but it had a lot of beds. And despite its relatively basic accommodations, many families preferred it because it was closer to their own homes. The nursing home itself did not make much of an impression on me. Meeting Jack Wilson did.

I accompanied the Grove's chaplain on a visit to Mr. Wilson. When we entered his room, we found him sitting in a chair, slumped over, eyes closed. The chaplain put his hand on Mr. Wilson's shoulder; he raised his head briefly and then put it down again. Mr. Wilson was blind and very hard of hearing. Communicating with him would take a little more than casual effort. The chaplain explained that Mr. Wilson needed an amplifying device to hear, but we did not see one in his room. After what felt like a very long ten minutes, we eventually found an aide who located his device in a drawer in the nurse's station. When we put the headphones on his ears, Mr. Wilson was a changed man. He and the chaplain had a simple yet cohesive conversation. He held my hand while I read a poem. Although we had never met, he smiled every time he heard my voice. Perhaps it was because I had the voice of a young woman. But it may have been more than that. From the aides to the nurses, nursing homes are filled with women's voices. I will never forget that smile nor our conversation, two things I had not thought him capable of when I first saw him, head bowed and eyes closed. I wondered how a man this sweet had ended up so alone.

I later learned that Mr. Wilson had not always been so sweet. He had struggled with alcohol most of his adult life. When he drank, he was reportedly not a very pleasant man. He had spent some parts of his adulthood on the streets and in homeless shelters. His inability to abstain from alcohol contributed to his inability to control the diabetes that took his vision. He had lived a hard life and had made life harder for everyone around him. He was a father of two but had not been much of a presence in their lives. In spite of this history, when he became old and frail, his oldest daughter had taken him in. The hoped-for family reconciliation was not to be. At his daughter's home, he used his network of friends to maintain his drinking habit. Moreover, he had not lost the tendency to rain down verbal and physical abuses when under its influence. He was eventually pushed out of the family circle. The nursing home was the only institution that stood between him and homelessness.

The Grove was never intended to replace unpaid family care. Its model relied on its ability to marshal family resources as well as organizational ones. The economic rationale of providing coordination and some amount of direct support is that it enables family members to provide unpaid care rather than relying on more expensive forms of state-funded care. However, the story of Mr. Wilson illustrates the challenges involved in making this a reality. Caring for a medically frail older adult is difficult under the best of circumstances. Many of the Grove's members did not live under the best of circumstances.

While reaching sixty-five moves many Americans into a protected economic class, they still enter this part of their lives with the same family dynamics, coping strategies, and orientation to their health as they held in midlife. Members like Mr. Wilson, who had difficulty parenting in youth or middle age, would often have adult children who not only struggled with their own economic and social vulnerabilities but also had conflicted relationships with their now-dependent parents. Failure to keep a member's network of survival active had consequences for the Grove. Adult children may have been motivated to keep their loved ones at home from a mix of affection and familial obligation, but for the Grove, there was an economic incentive. If the Grove could not keep a member living safely in the community, the member might have to transition to higher levels of care— the highest of which was nursing home residence. The Grove, however, remained administratively and financially responsible for member care, no matter the cost. Its capitation payments assumed financial responsibility until member-initiated disenrollment or death.

Because of this responsibility, the Grove needed cases like Mr. Wilson's to be aberrations. If partnership with a daughter, niece, or neighbor could keep members living in the community, the Grove had a better chance of remaining solvent. When the NPs helped members and their families manage problems with the Grove's own inefficiencies—smoothing over their frustrations as well as directly solving problems—they were not just assisting members and their families; they were helping the Grove control costs. By doing so, they were addressing the day-to-day solvency of the organization and playing a key role in the Grove's ability to demonstrate its utility to the state. The NPs may have had a professional stake in their performance of organizational care work. The Grove had an economic one.

The logic of interchangeability requires that NPs and physicians be held to account in the same ways. However, in my observations at the Grove, I saw more evidence of difference than of interchangeability. Both were hired for their medical expertise. Yet the NPs found themselves doing very different work from their physician colleagues. In part, this was attributable to their dissimilar orientations to patient care. Yet it seemed equally attributable to the dissimilar expectations of their employer. The NPs were pressed into becoming an organizational resource whose expertise was deployed by clinical staff and administrators. By contrast, attempts by staff to deploy the physicians' expertise were summarily rebuffed. The physicians retained the ability to autonomously define and control their own work, one of the chief prerequisites of professional status. In particular, they kept the scope of that work defined by their relationship to one client and one client only: the patient.

The Grove's administrators believed that these differences were a function of professional character. The NPs, they said, should learn to protect their time. If NPs were going to take on the work of physicians, they should learn to behave more like them than like nurses. Yet it is questionable whether the prerogatives of power are a matter of individual choice. The censure some NPs received when they tried to govern their own work revealed professional control to be a right seen as belonging to some occupations and not others. At the Grove, the difference between the NPs and physicians was partly a consequence of professional identity, but it was equally rooted in each group's relationship to their employer.

For the NPs, both patients and the Grove were clients to whom they had obligations. I argue that the dual obligation to patient and employer made their labor look less like medical work and more like care work. It was not just the content of the work that differed, but whom it was for. Scholars have observed that the relational nature of care work produces a sense of responsibility that is sometimes used by employers as a form of emotional labor. Emotional labor is defined as the efforts of workers to perform or feel certain emotions as a response to their employer's "feeling rules" (Hochschild 1983). While the work of managing and performing emotions is a ubiquitous part of social life, the concept of emotional labor specifically calls out its commercial deployment by employers. This deployment is not gender neutral. While people of all genders may be held accountable to feeling rules, women are more likely to be pressed into emotional labor because they disproportionally inhabit jobs where the performance of deference, friendliness, and nurturing is what employers desire. Even when women and men occupy the same jobs, colleagues and clients alike are more likely to hold women accountable to a gendered set of feeling rules (Cassell 1998; Davies 2003; Polletta and Tufail 2016).

The study of emotional labor has been fundamental to excavations of the invisibility of care work and its relationship to gendered expectations. The concept has illuminated the ways in which employers specifically benefit from the work as well as from its invisibility. However, the fruitfulness of this concept has, perhaps, been at the expense of exploring sites of hidden *material* work. Qualitative investigations of low-wage care workers suggest that an occupational identity rooted in caring for others produces not only emotional burdens but also the burdens of unremunerated work. Home care aides recount stories of working "off the clock" as well as taking on work for which they are unlicensed or that falls well beyond their assigned responsibilities (Stacey 2011, 2005). The hidden nature of the work is of value not only to these aides' clients but also to their employers. It is only because of this invisibility that employing agencies are able to retain clients whose care requirements would otherwise be unprofitable or outside their regulated scope of service.

At the Grove, what was invisible about the NPs' work was also of material value, both to members and to the organization. In some ways, the expansion of clinic concerns was part of the experimental nature of the entire organization. The Grove's mission of integrated care was premised on the idea that member problems did not have to fit within the narrow confines of a medical problem to be addressed. This mission was a tall organizational order that the Grove did not always meet. However, it was more likely to do so when its NPs took on these burdens from inside the clinic.

Employing organizations are a neglected client in much of the scholarship on medical professionals. Because of an almost exclusive focus on the case of physicians, health care organizations have been conceptualized primarily as a constraining force. Medicine's professional autonomy is measured, in part, by its ability to maintain a model of consultancy that protects its denizens from the meddling of organizations. They have been able to maintain this autonomy even in the face of significant structural changes in the industry. For example, the simple arithmetic of patients paying a fee for expert treatment has all but disappeared in modern heath care. Most physicians are paid through a series of organizational intermediaries in both the private and public sectors. Symbolically, however, their client remains the individual patient. Even when physicians work in health care organizations, they usually remain consultants. Anyone discharged from a hospital has had the experience of receiving one or more separate bills for these consultant services, in addition to their bill from the hospital. Physicians work in health care organizations, but they continue to resist being of them.

By contrast, professional nursing was shaped by its relationship with organizations. From its very inception, the growth and success of nursing was linked with the growth and success of the hospital. It is not happenstance that Florence Nightingale, the founding architect of the profession, was as much a hospital reformer as a professional empire builder (Holton 1984). For Nightingale, one of the chief roles of nursing was to bring order and cleanliness to what were chaotic and unhygienic hospital wards. Employed and deployed by hospitals, nursing work has always been a response to the needs of organizations, as much as to the direct needs of patients.

Intertwining its fate with the needs of bureaucratic health care organizations allowed nursing to expand its domain of work by demonstrating its utility. While the relationship between nursing and health care organizations has often been unbalanced—favoring the organization over the occupation—it has not been entirely one-sided. Organizations' ever-increasing need for skilled but inexpensive labor created seemingly infinite growth potential for nursing. Moreover, nurses' labor is reasonably well valued by the organizations that employ them. Both RNs and NPs make well over the US median salary.[1] When compared with the fate of other female-dominated professions, nursing's economic rewards are both singular and striking.

Nursing's responsibility for organizational concerns has continued to live on in contemporary professional claims (Allen 2014). After doing a review of published field studies of nursing work from 1993 to 2003, the scholar Davina Allen wrote, "It is nurses who reconcile the requirements of healthcare organisations with those of patients. . . . It is nurses who broker, interpret, translate and communicate clinical, social and organisational information in ways that are consequential for patient diagnoses and outcomes. It is nurses who work flexibly to blur their jurisdictional boundaries with those of others in order to ensure continuity of care. In fulfilling these roles, it is nurses who weave together the many facets of the service and create order in a fast flowing and turbulent work environment" (2004, 279).

When Norah described the NP as the "air traffic controller" of member needs, she was drawing on professionally salient notions of what nurses do. The work of coordination, and the demonstration of organizational utility, has remained a fundamental part of nursing work. While professional medicine still clings to a model of autonomous consultancy, professional nurses have always benefited from and been a benefit to health care organizations. At the Grove, I observed that the NPs were as much organizational actors as professional actors, called to be of use not only to patients but also to employers. Certainly, much of what they do remains hidden. It appeared that neither the Grove's members nor its staff were fully cognizant of what its NPs did, but they knew where to bring their concerns. As NPs continue to expand throughout US health care, they have the potential to make visible the need for and value of competent care work. We may simply have to pay more attention in order to see it.

Part II

A CHANGED TERRAIN FOR MEDICINE

NEW BOUNDARIES, NEW RELATIONSHIPS

Stanton School of Nursing often sponsored tours of the Grove. Physicians, nurses, and policy makers would come to learn about the Grove as both an innovative way to care for older adults and as an example of what nursing could achieve. Seven months into the position of medical director, Dr. Christine Morgan was asked to host such a tour along with Dean Kelly McCulloch, Stanton's administrative liaison with the Grove. As Christine recounted this story to me, she described a moment when Kelly was "going on and on about the nurse practitioners and how well they do what they do and the care that they provide." In the middle of this promotional narrative, one of the visitors asked a question. The questioner, Christine recalled, was a physician. "He was retired and doing research. But at his last position he had been the dean at Elite Medical School—so he was no slouch." He asked Kelly, "Well, if the nurse practitioners are the ones doing the majority of care, and everything is as you say, then why do you have a [physician] medical director?" Christine finished the story by saying, "I can't really remember Kelly's answer, but sometimes when you hear the way that she and others from Stanton talk about this place, you do wonder. There are people out in the community who don't realize that there are even physicians here."

The role of the physicians was a highly problematic question at the Grove. It was the obverse of what is usually problematized: the appropriate role of the NP. Stanton did not actively disparage the Grove's physicians. Indeed, the medical director had not been hidden away; she had been invited to participate in the tour. Yet Stanton had no clear vision for the role of professional medicine in its own world of nursing excellence. Policy makers often discuss NPs as if their presence were only about shifts in nursing: What should we allow NPs to do? In the aberrant world of the Grove, the unspoken question became the primary one: If nurses can assess, diagnose, and prescribe, what should the physicians be doing? The presence of the NP does not just signal changes in nursing work. It portends changes in medical work.

The shared boundary between the two professions has always been mutually constitutive. What it means to be a physician is not just defined by what physicians can do, but by what others, such as nurses, cannot (Allen 1997, 2000, 2001; Gieryn 1983; Norris 2001). Certainly, the work that lies on either side of the boundary has always been subject to change. The steady rise in nursing's status is undoubtedly linked with nurses' taking on work and responsibilities once held by physicians (Fairman and Lynaugh 2000; Sandelowski 2000). Professional medicine may not have always championed nursing's expansion, but it largely did not stand in the way—not so much because of its support of nurses, but because doing so served its own interests. The expansion of nursing work freed physicians to pursue work ever further removed from the immediacy of patient bodies, needs, and demands. The symbiotic quality of this relationship reveals a larger truth: although real tensions exist between nurses and physicians (Stein 1967; Stein, Watts, and Howell 1990), broadly speaking, they have worked collegially alongside one another for well over a century.

This collegiality has endured despite significant changes in what both physicians and nurses do for patients. Its endurance, however, has been predicated on the one thing that has not changed: the power relations between the two. While nursing has always claimed a separate but equal status with medicine, this assertion remains more ideal than reality. Physicians may not technically have authority over nurses; since the time of Nightingale, nursing has insisted on separate chains of command. But physician authority over the medical encounter has subordinated nursing nonetheless. Physicians have largely retained the cultural and institutional authority to control and direct all medical action, both physical and symbolic. Registered nurses may do a great deal more than carry out doctors' orders, but doing so is still part of the job. It is this difference in authority, and not just the difference in work, that undergirds the stability of the relationship between the two professions.

The NP threatens to disrupt that stability. When RNs become NPs, they are not just learning new skills; they are crossing lines of authority that they had previously learned to treat as constitutive of their profession (Trotter 2019). The nurse who wields authority in the medical encounter has been unsettling for both nursing and medicine. In this chapter, I look at the shape of that unsettling through the voices and experiences of NPs Norah, Michelle, and Anne. I found that their narrated and actual practices negotiated physician authority in very different ways. Although all voiced similar understandings of the different expertise physicians offered, each had worked out her own version of what it meant to be in right relationship with their physician colleagues. This variation created uncertainty for the physicians' understanding of their own work as well as for how the Grove organized the work of both providers.

The NP as Captain of the Ship

If time is the best teacher, NP Norah had enough under her belt to possess a clear sense of what it meant to be a nurse and an NP. When I met her, she had amassed over twenty years of NP experience, six of which had been at the Grove. She had a steady confidence in her own abilities and had little reticence in saying so. She was the NP who declared, "I'm good at what I do. And I think the Grove appreciates that." This confidence was reflected in how she described how she worked with physicians. She began by narrating the model of collaboration that nursing itself promotes. "In an ideal world it would be—and I've said it and I do mean it—I think the role of an NP and a physician should be synergistic rather than separate. Together even stronger." I have no reason to doubt that she did, in fact, mean it. But by her own admission, there was a contradiction between this ideal and reality. In describing her own approach, she was quite candid. "This is terrible, but I guess I look at [the physicians] for me personally as almost like consultants rather than collaborators. I grab them when I'm stuck." Norah was aware of the contradiction, almost seeming to apologize. Yet she made no apologies for how she cared for her members. When Norah entered the doors of the clinic, she did so, unapologetically, as the captain of her own ship.

At the Grove, Norah was the NP for whom the theme of autonomy and clinical independence was most salient. It was the lack of autonomy in other forms of nursing that had motivated her to become an NP. Norah began her nursing career as a bedside nurse. At twenty-one years old and fresh out of university, she had entered the ranks of hospital RNs. Acute care hospitals remain the primary employer of RNs in the US; it is not surprising that this was where she found her first job. "In the beginning," she said, "it was a great job." However, the glow of her chosen career began to dim after the first year. "It wasn't that I didn't like it. I mean, I liked the patients; I loved the people I worked with." For Norah, the main problem was not the nursing work; it was everything else. "There was a lot of stuff that I was being judged on that wasn't really nursing related." She recalled being held responsible for making sure the rooms were clean and the trash was emptied. "I don't want to say I was a glorified maid. But you really don't have a lot of autonomy. You don't have a lot of say. You don't have a lot of control. You just have to follow orders. And that's not what I wanted to do."

Norah's desire to move away from hospital nursing represents a common experience. The unrelenting pace and physical nature of the job push many to pursue less taxing, if lower-paid, nursing positions outside the hospital, especially as they age (Auerbach, Buerhaus, and Staiger 2014). Norah considered going into nursing administration—a well-trodden path taken by nurses hoping to "get off the floor"—but what she liked most about nursing was providing direct patient care. She did not want to move away from the bedside; she simply wanted a different way to be there. Unlike previous generations of nurses, Norah had an alternative option. She could become an NP.

In the 1980s, the population of NPs was still quite small; the best estimates suggest that there were twenty-two thousand (Ostwald and Abanobi 1986). As a matter of nursing education, however, the NP was fully institutionalized when Norah began to consider her next steps (Brush and Capezuti 1996). When Norah attended an open house at Stanton School of Nursing, the route to becoming an NP was well laid out. She did not have to be a pioneer; she simply had to enroll. Going to school part-time, she was able to finish a master's of science in nursing (MSN) in three years, specializing in geriatric care.

Her first NP position took her as far away from the hospital as one could possibly get. She accepted a job within a home care practice that provided incontinence management for older adults. Norah relished working outside the regimentation of the hospital hierarchy. Moreover, the practice was owned and operated by two NPs, making her feel more like a colleague than a hired hand. She enjoyed the position, but after seven years, she found herself "getting bored" because it was all urology. "I was only there for one thing. And that's when I realized I really wanted to get more into primary care."

In 1998, she found the opportunity to do just that at Sunshine Pavilion, a retirement community that offered medical and supportive care. In the years she worked at the Pavilion, Norah not only expanded her clinical skills; she also solidified her own view of what it meant to work alongside physicians. She went from working in an NP-only practice to one where there was a significant physician presence. Yet this presence was paired with an absence constituted by segregation. The Pavilion had no organizational philosophy of teamwork. When she was working, the physicians often were not. Norah explained, "I worked with two physicians who were only there part-time. So for the most part—probably 60 percent of the time—I was the most experienced medical person there on site." Even when they overlapped in time, they did not overlap in space.

"The physicians worked with me, but I had my caseload, basically, and they had theirs. There are some people that they never saw because I saw them all."

At the Pavilion, where NPs and physicians did not meet in the same space or share the same patients, an everyday reliance on physician input would have been at odds with the practical requirements of the job. In this context, Norah had developed a model of consultancy rather than collaboration. Casting the physicians as consultants required an acknowledgment that they possessed expertise that she did not. Without prompting from me, Norah declared her recognition of that expertise. "There's a lot of things that [the physicians] understand *way* better than I do." Yet one can acknowledge that a consultant has different expertise without accepting a subordinate status. Norah continued, "I think where NPs excel is in the treatment of chronic illness. Once we know what the established chronic problem is, I think the NP's role is ideal in managing that chronic problem. But the front end of figuring out what [the problem] is? . . . I think that's where the physicians really excel." Norah trusted the physicians to do what they did well, but was confident in her ability to independently excel as an NP. As Norah continued to describe her ideal relationship, it became clear that her different-but-equal model required mutual recognition. It was not enough for Norah to recognize the physicians' expertise; they had to recognize that she had her own. At the Pavilion, Norah believed she had that recognition. In describing her relationship with the Pavilion's physicians, she noted, "I had a very good relationship with both of them. They trusted me; I trusted them. They knew I would call them if there was a problem."

This was the model that Norah had developed at the Pavilion, and it was the one she brought with her when she joined the Grove in 2005. This model, however, was a less-than-easy fit for the Grove. The fundamental difference between the Pavilion and the Grove was their patient populations. As a privately funded facility, the Pavilion was a luxury good. Its residents had the economic resources to retire comfortably, and they entered old age with the social stability and better health that are associated with those resources. The Grove's members had many fewer of their own resources and relied more heavily on publicly funded, organizational ones. Moreover, as a nursing home diversion program, the Grove systematically selected for members who were prone to medical instability and who lived with significant impairments.

The NPs were the first to acknowledge the clinical challenge of working at the Grove. Norah distinctly recalled her reaction when she first started treating the Grove's members. "It was like holy crap; these people are bad!" She was seeing women and men at the tail end of their lives with conditions such as end stage renal disease, end stage congestive heart failure, and chronically uncontrolled diabetes and hypertension. Physician acknowledgment of NP expertise might be less forthcoming in an environment in which the required expertise was fairly high. The Grove, however, would prove to be challenging in a way that was unexpected. At the Grove, Norah had to grapple with physician proximity in a way she never had before. Her NP career had largely excluded the experience of working for, or even largely working with, a physician. Ironically, it was not until she took a position at a self-identified nurse-managed practice that she experienced the possibility of true physician collaboration. Out of that possibility, she had her first encounters with physician resistance.

The Physician as Consultant

Dr. Jeremy Simons was one of the physicians on staff when Norah began working at the Grove. He spent some mornings doing rounds at the hospital, but more than half his time was spent in the clinic. Norah's view of the physician as a consultant did not sit well with Jeremy. "He made it very clear to me that he was irritated that I never communicated with him. He really wanted to know what was going on and he got visibly angry with me. He would start grinding his teeth together, saying, 'You really don't like me to know what's going on, do you Norah.' And no, it wasn't that; it's just that I didn't think he needed to know.... They were *my* people. They were *my* members. They were *my* patients."

Casting the physician as consultant may not seem to call for a literal gnashing of teeth. After all, the role of physician-consultant is entrenched throughout the US health care system. Although patients are increasingly referring themselves to specialists of their own choosing, many—either by choice or by their insurance providers' decrees—continue to rely on primary care providers to decide when to seek specialty care. This gatekeeping role is not just an administrative function; it is a professional one. While acknowledging that patients require someone else's expertise, referring providers are entrusted with the responsibility of knowing when they have reached the borders of their own. No one is looking over referring physicians' shoulders; they make their own decisions.

Herein lay the source of conflict between Norah's vision of consultancy and its typical formulation. In the traditional model of consultancy, the referring provider does not send over a task or a problem, but a person. The consult is for the client, and the client is the patient. When the physicians were recast as consultants for the NPs, it was not they who determined when they were needed or often what was needed; it was the NPs. This shift in who guides the action suggests a more radical change than first appears. In Norah's model of consultancy, it was almost as if she had become the physician's client. The physician was asked to address her questions rather than the direct concerns of patients.

This model of consultancy may not produce conflict at organizations like the Pavilion, where physicians and NPs are separated by time and geography. At the Grove, however, these two types of clinicians found themselves working in shared terrain with shared patients. In this setting, the client-like demands of the NPs reshaped the physicians' work in unaccustomed ways. "[The physicians] were feeling like their job was just to sit around and wait until we said 'I don't know what to do about this, that, or the other thing.'" This was the observation of NP Francesca. She was recounting a set of meetings between the NPs and physicians that had happened in 2009, before my fieldwork began. During those meetings, the NPs learned that Jeremy's teeth-grinding was less about what Norah was doing and more about what he was not. Both he and the medical director flatly rejected the model of physician as consultant. Francesca summarized, "[The NPs] didn't know how much the physicians wanted to have regular member contact. We thought they were happy being 'out there' some place."

I could not ask the previous physicians about their preferred model for working with the NPs, but I could ask the current ones. Their rejection of the physician-as-consultant model was communicated through their descriptions of their ideal relationship with the NPs. Dr. Tracy Polson believed that NPs and physicians "could share the work," but that physicians were best suited as the primary decision makers for medical care. Dr. Renee Michaels used much stronger terms. She described her ideal relationship with the NPs in this way: "[The NPs] practice within their scope of comfort. And then go to their supervising physician and say, 'This is what I did and I think it's fine. Or this is what I did, and I don't know what to do next.'" Renee had no administrative title at the Grove. Yet she described herself as the "supervising physician" of any NP with whom she worked. Renee explicitly used the word "supervising" in regard to the NPs, while Tracy did not. But each described an ideal in which the NP was skilled and helpful, but was a clear subordinate. Their ideal relationship looked a lot less like consultancy and more like the relationship between an attending physician and a resident. Attendings *are* supervisors. No matter how knowledgeable or skilled a resident might be, the attending remains the captain of the ship.

The assertion that physicians should retain their customary role as captains puts the Grove's physicians in line with the prevailing view of their profession's advocates. For organizations such as the AMA, the NP as captain is a polite fiction at best; at worst, it is a subterfuge that emboldens nursing at the expense of patient care. In addition to legislative moves to block NP independence, the AMA has made rhetorical moves to rewrite the NP as a minor addition to the traditional medical hierarchy. The AMA has referred to the NP as a "physician support occupation" and argues that NPs should only work "under the direct supervision or direction" of physicians (2005). Norah's model of consultancy was categorically at odds with the one put forward by the AMA and the Grove's physicians. Her model, however, was not the only one in circulation at the Grove.

The NP as Second-in-Command

NP Michelle had a very different orientation from Norah, to both her practice and her relationship with physicians. When I asked Michelle to describe what an NP is, she responded, "At nurse practitioner school we're taught to recognize what's normal. . . . Okay, I don't know what this is but it's not normal. So let me confer. Or let me look it up. It's like primary care docs refer to rheumatologists. Well, nurse practitioners refer to medical docs." Michelle seemed to be invoking the physician as consultant. In practice, however, I observed that her version of consulting came closest to the AMA's view of the physician as captain of the ship. In her everyday work in the clinic, Michelle seemed most comfortable inhabiting the role of second-in-command.

Michelle and Norah shared the same physician: Tracy. Yet their interactions with her were strikingly dissimilar. Even though Tracy's office was in Norah's alcove, the two of them could go days without sharing more than a friendly "good morning." By contrast, Michelle would visit Tracy as a routine part of her day. Her preferred practice was to gather her thoughts, usually at the end of a clinic day, and walk over to Tracy's office. There, she would share changes in member medications, abnormal lab work, and updates on member care. Although Michelle sometimes asked specific clinical questions, these conversations were not purely consultative. In addition to case reports, she also shared much of the contextual information that she had learned from and about members throughout the day. Michelle treated Tracy not just as a clinical resource for what she could do for her patients, but as someone with whom she actively shared member care. Because their offices were in different locations, these were not chance encounters. Michelle had to make a special trip in order to facilitate these conversations. No physicians complained about Michelle's failure to communicate. If it had been up to her, she would have done so on a daily basis.

In some respects, Michelle's relationship with Tracy looked like the model of collaboration that Norah described as her ideal, if not actual, practice. But Michelle's enactment of collaboration was a one-way street. Tracy got along well with Michelle and seemed to genuinely enjoy her company. Both had been working in health care longer than almost anyone else at the Grove; their closeness in age seemed to bring them together. They had a very collegial relationship, but it was not exactly an equal one. I never witnessed Tracy making any pilgrimages to Michelle's office to share her own thoughts about members.

Collaboration between the two depended entirely on Michelle's initiative. Michelle came closest to the kind of NP that the AMA says it wants. She was skilled and conscientious. But she made a concerted effort to run all significant medical decisions by a physician. The physician remained the captain, while the NP acted on her behalf.

Michelle's embodiment as the second-in-command can be more deeply understood in the context of her own career biography. Michelle had a long nursing career before coming to the Grove. But when she first entered nursing, it looked very different than it does now. Michelle graduated from a Catholic high school in 1957, a time when there were few professional career opportunities for women. Michelle described herself as a curious student. She knew she wanted to do something after high school, but college was not an option. "I come from a family where we weren't really poor but we didn't have extra money. . . . I liked medicine. But college I just viewed as not being for me." She recalled that her high school guidance counselor had advised that she could either "be a teacher or a nurse." She chose nursing.

Michelle entered a hospital-based, vocational diploma program. One nurse described such programs as akin to an apprenticeship "because you worked in the hospital after your first six months." Diploma programs rather than university schooling were the most salient form of nursing education well into the 1970s, making nursing both affordable and accessible to a large population of women. Throughout much of the twentieth century, nursing provided one of the only opportunities for "respectable work" for women who either wanted or needed paid employment. This career option was particularly valuable for women on the lower end of the economic spectrum. For Michelle, this accessibility informed her choice more than inspiration. Her mother cashed in a life insurance policy for one thousand dollars; this investment was all she needed to pay for three years of training and to start her career.

If Michelle lived through what nursing once was, she also lived through what nursing has since become. In pursuit of higher status, nursing sought to trade in its vocational diplomas for university degrees. In 1965, the American Nurses' Association publicly declared its position that the bachelor's of science in nursing (BSN) should be the standard of entry to nursing (1965). This pronouncement was neither law nor regulation, but it did begin to influence the choices of prospective nurses and their employers. Even as Michelle neared the end of her diploma program, she was advised, "'You really need to get your BSN.' . . . Well, that was back in the sixties. And [the BSN] is *still* not required. But the bug was in the ear: you have to get your BSN." Nine years after she received her RN license, Michelle began taking classes part-time toward the degree. It took her a little longer than she planned because she got married and had two children along the way. But she successfully earned her BSN in 1974. Becoming an NP, however, would be a much longer road.

In the 1970s, the NP role was so new that it was not a commonly known option. Michelle had already found a path away from hospital nursing by becoming a nurse educator. But as nursing transitioned toward university-based training, her BSN was no longer enough to qualify her to continue teaching. It was while she was investigating master's programs that Michelle discovered the NP. Even then, she stumbled upon the option only after starting a different course of study. She had begun taking classes toward an MSN as a clinical nurse specialist. Clinical nurse specialists are master's-trained nurses who also care for patients, but they were created for inpatient rather than outpatient settings and thus do not have the same level of practice independence as NPs.[1] Michelle remembers the day she met her first NP. She was taking an elective called Aging in Society, which was taught by a social worker and an NP. As she learned more about what the NP did, she remembers thinking, "That is so neat what this nurse practitioner is doing. That's what I should do. I'll be a nurse practitioner." She changed her course of study and never looked back.

At the age of forty-nine, Michelle became a geriatric NP. Although the NP was created for the outpatient setting, she found her first NP job in the hospital, providing care for older adults who were awaiting discharge. In many ways, the job was a good fit for her years of experience in the hospital. At the time, however, the role of the NP in the acute care setting was still experimental. Her job responsibilities were constantly in flux, and over time, they slowly began to shrink. Her work began looking less and less like that of the NP she had worked so hard to become. Although she stayed at the hospital for almost twenty years, she eventually concluded that moving on was the best thing to do. As a consequence of luck or fate, her decision to leave coincided with an opening at the Grove.

For Michelle, the move to the Grove was an opportunity to challenge herself, professionally and clinically. She had never worked in an outpatient setting. And she had never served as a patient's primary care provider. The Grove was the chance to see what it felt like to really be in charge. Given her lack of experience in primary care, she fully expected to learn on the job. This was not an unreasonable expectation. Despite nursing's professional aspirations, it continues to have one foot in its vocational past. It remains a salient notion that "any nurse can be trained to do any nursing activity," even within the NP labor market. When Michelle arrived, she was aware that there were things she had to learn about primary care. "It was a stretch for me because I had all these years of not doing it. And it was hard." She knew it would be a challenge, but she also anticipated that she'd have help. She was confident in her ability to distinguish normal from abnormal, but she expected the physician to have the final word on treatment. She had no problem being second-in-command when it came to medical decision-making. The only difficulty with this approach is that it required physician presence. At times, this was in short supply.

When the Captain Is Hard to Find

When the current cohort of physicians arrived at the Grove, there was a lot of experimenting with how best to incorporate them into the clinic. At first, the physicians moved to embed themselves more deeply into routine member care. Once there were enough physicians to do so, they organized themselves by team affiliation. Although any physician might be turned to in an emergency, a stable team identity provided an opportunity for the physicians to become familiar with a panel of members—to really be a part of the team. When Tracy arrived, she had suggested that the physicians and NPs alternate the mandated six-month assessments. These comprehensive assessments were fairly time intensive. For the NPs, having the physicians share the burden was both of practical help and a structural nod to the kind of team-based collaboration the NPs said they wanted. Not only were "two eyes better than one," but also members would have the clinical benefit of being seen by providers with different strengths. It was a decision that both the physicians and the NPs supported. This was the kind of synergy that Norah referenced as nursing's ideal: "together even stronger."

Despite their initial impulse to integrate themselves into the clinic, the physicians soon began finding the work outside it more appealing. There had always been a certain amount of clinical work to be done outside the Grove's walls. Part of how the Grove supports its members is by providing continuity of care. On any given day, there were members being admitted to or discharged from the hospital. There were always a certain number of members who resided, temporarily or long term, within a nursing home. The Grove had to manage the care of its members no matter where they were located. This presented both a practical and a professional problem for the NPs.

At the time of my fieldwork, it was unusual for NPs to have hospital privileges. The Grove's NPs would sometimes visit members in the hospital, but without privileges, they could not do any of the formal work required. The role of NPs at nursing homes was a bit more varied. Before the Grove had its current triad of physicians, the NPs completed the six-month medical assessments for nursing home residents, but the physicians did the day-to-day work of following resident care. One NP explained that most nursing homes are "really funny about NPs coming in there and writing orders." In effect, the NPs provided the aspects of care mandated by the Grove, and the physicians did the work required by the nursing home. Perhaps because of the logic of how the work was divided, the NPs still considered the members in nursing homes as *their* members. The NPs were still their primary care providers and felt responsible for their care. That was the status quo until the new physicians decided that things needed to change.

At one primary care meeting, a weekly meeting with NPs and physicians, Christine notified the NPs of the change in policy. The physicians had decided that it would be more efficient if they took over clinical responsibility for the members in nursing homes. The reasoning was straightforward: when nursing homes wanted patient information or signed orders, it made sense to have one person fielding those requests rather than sometimes an NP and sometimes a physician. From a practical perspective, if physicians were already traveling to nursing homes, it seemed reasonable for them to complete the six-month assessments. Upon hearing this decision, the NPs had varying points of view about its benefits. Some NPs had struggled to manage the care of nursing home residents with their in-clinic work. For them, it was a relief to hand that responsibility over to someone else. For others, the loss of their relationships with nursing home residents was a significant one. Whatever its merits, this change would signal more than an administrative shift in who did what. It proved to be the first of many steps the physicians would take to move their work out of the clinic.

With each passing day, the physicians seemed to spend more of their time at the hospital and nursing home and less time at the Grove. Even when they were on site, there were meetings and paperwork to attend to in parts of the Grove other than the clinic. Their investment in member care remained high, but their investment in the clinic seemed to disappear. The physicians did not, as a practice, make themselves dependably available for face-to-face contact. No one ever knew when a particular physician would be physically present in the clinic. When a clinic receptionist or aide would ask an RN or NP about the whereabouts of Renee or Tracy, there would be an ambiguous shrug followed by, "I think she's at the nursing home." Without a regular and dependable presence, the physicians remained only peripheral figures in the clinic.

The NPs had been more than ready to share their work with the physicians. Instead, the physicians found new work, leaving the NPs to manage clinic concerns on their own. As these physicians moved more and more of their practice away from the clinic, The model of second-in-command would become increasingly difficult to live out. Daily reliance on physicians' input required their presence. Yet the physicians were increasingly absent. And as physicians more generally absent themselves from primary care, Michelle's version of collaboration may prove less sustainable than Norah's model of consultancy.

The NP as Team Player

In contrast to Norah and Michelle, NP Anne saw herself as neither captain nor second-in-command but as part of a team with shared responsibility. This "middle of the road" approach is in line with her own career biography. In terms of chronology, Anne's experience in nursing resides somewhere in between those of Michelle and Norah. Like Michelle, becoming an NP was something she chose fairly late in her nursing career. She had already worked fifteen years as a nurse before she became a geriatric NP. She had been working in health care even longer. After high school, she had taken a job as a hospital clerk at Franklin Hospital. But she knew she wanted more than a job; she wanted a career. In the early 1970s, there were not many career options available for women; even fewer for those who did not attend college. As with Michelle, nursing would turn out to be a good choice in part because it was an attainable choice. Going to school while she worked, she trained for her first nursing credential via an associate's degree. Although this path is less common today, an associate's degree still qualifies one to sit for the RN licensing exam.

Deciding to stay on at Franklin Hospital, she transitioned from clerk to nurse. But after two years at the bedside, Anne began looking for a way out. Like Norah, she knew "that the last thing I wanted to do was stay working on the floor." But unlike Norah, becoming an NP was not yet part of her universe of choices. Instead, she chose the more common path of moving into administration. That path would require a university degree. State nursing boards make no distinction between the nursing work performed by those with associate's degrees and that performed by bachelor's degree holders, but the state is not the only evaluator of nursing skill.[2] As part of the goal of raising its status, the nursing profession has continued to press for university training as the standard for all nurses. While hospitals have not accepted this call with quite the speed the profession would have liked, they often do place a higher value on bachelor's-trained nurses.

Anne had good reason to believe that without a college degree, she would have difficulty qualifying for positions away from the bedside. Earning a few credits at a time, she finished her BSN at the age of thirty-one. Armed with her new degree, she "started applying for everything that came down the pike, management-wise." She eventually landed a position in staff development, coordinating the hospital's internal nursing training and continuing education programs. Anne enjoyed her new position; she also credits it with introducing her to the field of nursing education. As she hoped, her new degree moved her off the floor.

Anne's career was marked by upward transitions in much the same way as the nursing profession. Every time she looked for a new opportunity, nursing was half a step ahead. When Anne earned her BSN in 1982, the NP was still a fledgling provider. In the hospital setting, where Anne had spent her entire working life, NPs were virtually nonexistent. So when she began considering her next professional move, it was not to become an NP but, like Michelle, to become a clinical nurse specialist. Anne hoped to use her MSN in the same way that she had used her BSN: to move up in the hospital hierarchy.

While continuing to work full-time, Anne began taking a few classes at Stanton School of Nursing. It was there that she first learned about NPs. "I was at Stanton probably six months. I was in class and somebody said, 'You must be one of those nurse practitioner students.' And I said, 'A what?'" Having spent her entire career in the same hospital, she had not encountered anything as exotic as an NP. "We had [no NPs] in our hospital. I'd basically grown up there . . . as a unit clerk, got my associate's, became a staff nurse, got my bachelor's, came to staff development. I was there for a total of thirteen years. So that was all I knew."

Anne decided to learn more about the NP role. What she discovered made her change course. "I thought, well, this will make me more marketable in the long run. . . . While [all nurses with master's degrees] are called advanced practice nurses, clinical specialists cannot prescribe. I thought well, becoming an NP, I'll have another license. I can teach because [being an NP] doesn't preclude you from teaching. But I could also hang out my shingle and be independent. I could work with a doctor. I could work in a variety of settings. And so it was dumb luck. Best dumb luck I ever had." Three and a half years later, she graduated from Stanton as an NP. Once Anne had her master's degree and NP license, she used these new credentials to continue fashioning a career. As a geriatric NP, she worked in nursing homes, assisted living facilities, and inside the hospital, but never in outpatient primary care. It was never something she thought she would do—until she began teaching NP students.

As a nursing instructor, part of her job was to assess her students' clinical skills during their rotations. That was when she realized she wanted a change. "I was sitting in these doctors' offices, and it was like I had to keep sitting on my hands—figuratively—just to keep my mouth shut. I really wanted to take care of the patients." Anne did not have to go looking for that chance; it came looking for her. "I'll never forget, it was a Wednesday night. It was right around four thirty, and I see this email come through that there's an opening for an NP at the Grove. Please consider applying for it." She didn't expect to get the job when she applied. She had a lot of NP experience, but she had never worked in primary care. But when she got the offer, she said yes.

That she got the job was unexpected, but not improbable. Like Michelle, Anne was accustomed to the idea of learning on the job. The opportunity to learn was one of the attractions of the position. Anne knew she would learn a lot from the Grove's NPs, but she also anticipated learning from the physicians. Physician mentorship remains an explicit part of NP training. Even in many of the states where NPs have gained full practice autonomy, there is a mandated waiting period of six months to a year when direct physician supervision is required.

Formal regulation aside, newly trained NPs often have an expectation of physician mentorship at their first NP positions.

During my fieldwork at Stanton School of Nursing, I listened to students describe "good" first jobs versus "bad" first jobs. The distinction between the two relied primarily on physician mentorship. A good job was, as one student noted, "where the doctor really understands that I'm a new nurse practitioner. They have to be willing to train me." Students told cautionary tales of bad first jobs where an NP was thrown into a practice "where the doc wouldn't even be there." When Anne started at the Grove, she was certainly not a new NP, but she was new to the kind of work she would be asked to do. That Anne would need clinical mentoring was not a secret. But for the physicians to fill this need, they had to be both present and willing to mentor. Anne found some physicians more willing to do so than others.

Sharing Medical Responsibility

When Anne joined the Grove in 2008, the medical director was Dr. Sean Martin. He inhabited this role on a part-time basis; he had another position at a large health system and was only sporadically available at the Grove. As the medical director, if anyone could be said to supervise the NPs' clinical practice, it would have been him. Although Anne never used the word "supervise" in this context, she did assume that Sean would play some role as a clinical mentor in helping her transition to primary care. However, this assumption was more of a hope than a certainty, because for Anne, Sean was not an unknown quantity.

When she was an NP student, one of Anne's last clinical rotations was with Sean. She was placed with him in order to learn the practice of primary care within the home—the modern version of the physician home visit. She recalled that she met with him on the first day of her placement and he promptly handed her off to the RNs on staff, never to be seen again. Instead of learning new skills, Anne spent that rotation filling a nursing position, using skills she already possessed. "Sean was my precept; I was supposed to be seeing patients with him. . . . Why he bothered to take a student I don't know, but he didn't want to be bothered." When Anne got to the Grove, she quickly surmised that "he basically hadn't changed in twenty years. . . . He never mentored me when I was a student. And he didn't mentor me when I was a new person here."

Anne's story of Sean's unavailability was not a general critique about how he did his job as the medical director. By most accounts, he was well respected by almost everyone at the Grove; even Anne had no specific qualms about his leadership. Instead, her criticism was about how his absence negatively impacted her practice as an NP. Anne specifically used the word "mentor" to describe what she wanted in a physician. She was not looking for someone to simply make decisions beyond her ken; she wanted someone to help her learn to make better ones. As Anne reflected on her experiences at the Grove after three years, she noted, "Now, I actually feel fairly comfortable in this position. Not totally. There are still a few things where I hit a brick wall. I'm not a doc. I'm a nurse practitioner. But I feel comfortable adjusting hypertension meds and diabetes meds. These are all things I didn't know. . . . I can do it now. But that transition was hard." For Anne, the physicians who helped her make that transition were better colleagues than those who did not. But clinical mentoring was not the only ideal she wanted the physicians to embody. She wanted a teammate; someone to work with. She believed she had found that in Renee.

During my fieldwork, Renee was the full-time physician assigned to Anne's team. Anne described her experience with Renee in the following way: "She knows the members. I can go and talk to her about something and she can come talk to me about something and we can banter back and forth about, 'well, did you try this, how's this going, did you—what's this diagnostic, what happened with that, what's the next step in the process.' That to me is collaborative, and that's the first time I've experienced it." She compared her relationship with Renee with one of the previous physicians, recounting, "If I had a problem that I couldn't solve as the NP, I'd go to the physician. I presented the case as if I was a resident. And they'd say, 'Oh, did you try blah blah blah?' They never again ask me, 'Did you try it? Did it work? How's the patient now?' . . . So there was no carryover, there was no investment in the patient. Which, I'm not saying that's a bad thing or a good thing, it's just an observation. It was purely consultative. . . . There was no investment in the particular team."

Anne knew and accepted her role as the leader of the team. Yet her preferred vision of leadership was not a solo endeavor. She preferred to think of her members as shared terrain. They were "our members" as much as they were "my members." When she described what was dissatisfying about her previous physician relationships, she noted, "What I found was that I was in charge of all the patients. I was responsible for all the follow-up. I was the leader of the team. I still am. But I was up there *all by myself*." Anne did not just want someone with whom to share the work; she wanted someone with whom to share the responsibility.

Anne's team-player model would seem to have the best of both worlds. But this approach shared some of the same drawbacks as Michelle's model. At a fundamental level, it required physician presence. Although it did not require the same level of presence as the second-in-command model, it required more physician investment, not only in patient care but also in the NP's professional development. In the second-in-command approach, the investment required was all on the part of the NP. Michelle took the initiative to collaborate with the physician. She was the one who made her way to the physician's office. She was the one who gathered her thoughts together in order to ask the physician specific questions. Michelle may not have taken total responsibility for making medical decisions, but in her own way, she took complete responsibility for getting them made. In Anne's ideal, the physician had to independently perform investment in and responsibility for member care. It was not enough for a physician to offer a recommendation. Anne wanted someone who would return to ask, "Did it work?" It is unclear, however, how well Anne's model of shared responsibility can work within our current framework for health care delivery.

There was a case early on in my fieldwork in which one of the Grove's members had high prostate-specific antigen (PSA) values for several years, an indication of prostate cancer. These values had been noted by one of the physicians. In his clinical notes, the physician documented that follow-up was needed. From his perspective, that was the extent of his responsibility. Acting as a consultant, he had written his expert opinion. The member had an NP as his primary care provider; she had the responsibility for following up. However, the member's NP (whose pseudonym I am intentionally omitting) had not taken on this responsibility. From the NP's perspective, the physician had performed the exam; he would take responsibility for making sure that follow-up occurred. When it did not, there were questions about what had gone wrong and who was at fault.

From my view as a sociologist, there was plenty of blame to go around. The Grove, it seemed to me, bore some responsibility for helping its clinicians develop effective systems of communication in a mandated team environment. However, one of the Grove's nurses reminded me that health care is not the place for theorizing. Speaking to me about the case, this RN opined that, as the primary care provider, the NP had been the one in charge. In the hierarchical world of medicine, responsibility goes straight to the top. If being in charge was what an NP wanted, it did not matter what anyone else did or did not do; the buck stopped with her.

Shared responsibility is an ideal that is difficult to live out in an industry where the threat of lawsuits holds material consequences for being the one in charge. Underneath abstractions like "the team" and "collaboration," health care is still organized around the assumption that someone is in charge and that someone is responsible when things go wrong. In this context, responsibility cannot really be shared, at least not in the way that some NPs might desire.

At the Grove, as well as in US health care more broadly, the physicians that NPs are replacing are still very much here. Despite their migration into specialty practice, physicians still represent 70 percent of the primary care work force (Agency for Healthcare Research and Quality 2012). This macro-level presence is reflected at the micro level. According to a recent survey, 89 percent of NPs work in a setting with at least some physician presence, with 56 percent reporting that a physician was present at their practice at least 75 percent of the time (Health Resource and Services Administration 2014). Nurse practitioners may find themselves needing to dually negotiate physician presence *and* absence. This dual negotiation not only raises the question of how NPs and physicians will work together but how they will carve up the terrain of patient problems and clinical responsibility.

At the Grove, these questions had more than one answer. Norah, Michelle, and Anne were all practicing in the same state, working for the same employer, and asked to treat patients with the same level of complexity. However, each had crafted a distinct orientation to practice which incorporated the physicians in different ways. The resources used to craft these orientations were not idiosyncratic but came out of nursing's own history of change. As evidenced through their career biographies, nursing education and credentialing regimes have changed dramatically in the last seven decades. The nonstandard nature of state regulations and employer protocols adds to the variability of NP practice. Nurse practitioners who move across state lines, or even just change jobs, may find themselves inhabiting an expanded or reduced role irrespective of their own experience or competence. If NP practices are partly a function of the professional biographies such regimes produce, then the question of what NPs should do will have more than one answer for some time to come.

In some ways, the uncertainty surrounding NP practice has proved to be an opportunity for nursing. The swirl of educational and credentialing change has sometimes opened the door for NPs and their employers to provide new answers to the question of what NPs can do. This uncertainty created room for Michelle to spend a fifty-year career growing into an autonomous provider and a fifty-year-old Norah to become, as one NP colleague called her, "the best nurse practitioner I've ever met in my whole life." The Grove too was a place where NPs stretched the boundaries of nursing expertise. Having the opportunity to provide and manage care for a medically fragile population was a challenging but rewarding experience for the NPs I followed. In this regard, they are not unique. It is a fairly open secret that NPs, once envisioned to only be suitable for preventive care and minor illness, are increasingly deployed to care for those with the highest burdens of illness and the most complicated medical needs (DesRoches et al. 2017; Diers and Molde 1983).

This uncertainty may have created opportunity for nurses, but it has produced an existential crisis for physicians. When NPs cross the boundary between nursing and medicine, we should expect effects beyond the personnel arithmetic of employers. It is not just task allocation or work that constitutes these boundaries, but deeper questions of identity and meaning. Who NPs consider themselves to be is not just an internal matter, but one that has implications for physician identity as well as the broader organization of health care. The physicians who worked with Norah were expected to sit around until she asked for help. Those who worked with Michelle could expect daily consultations, and those who worked with Anne were expected to be independently invested in both patient care and NP mentoring. At the Grove, these different demands were especially problematic because they were being made on the same people. The same physician might be expected to captain one ship and leave another alone. The physicians were pressured to be what each NP needed, rendering the NP both colleague and client.

Individualized notions of NP practice also raise questions for how employers should organize the work. The true paradox among the Grove's NPs was that although none expressed the ideal of the physician as consultant, this was the model that seemed to best serve the needs of the organization because it required the least amount of physician investment. As a matter of historical record, the existence of the NP was premised on the reality of physician disinvestment. Between 1985 and 2011, the proportion of US medical students who chose primary care residencies declined by 24 percent. Moreover, between 1999 and 2003, the proportion of internal medicine residents who went on to work in primary care dropped from 54 percent to 20 percent (Schwartz 2012). By contrast, the proportion of NPs trained in primary care remains high. In 2018, an estimated 87 percent of NPs reported a primary care area as their main specialty (American Association of Nurse Practitioners 2019). When nursing organizations marshal arguments for NP practice independence, they cite such evidence to demonstrate NPs' willingness to be present in the face of physician absence. Forecasts of physician shortages legitimated the creation of the NP in the 1960s; fifty years later, a set of similarly dire predictions anchor claims for NP expansions in work and autonomy. The utility of the NP is lessened if physician presence is still required.

Norah may have been the Grove's idealized NP not only because she solved a wide variety of patient and organizational problems but also because her practice of treating the physician as a consultant was the best match for an organization operating under a field-level set of constraints that includes physician scarcity. Two and a half years after she started, Renee decided to leave the Grove. In response to organizational murmurings about hiring a physician to replace her, Christine sent an email to all staff which said that they had an advertisement out, but full-time geriatricians were difficult to find. Other practices in the city maintained unfilled vacancies for years. She had no expectation that they would find anyone soon. The clinic would likely be down a physician for some time to come.

5

GAINING STATUS, LOSING GROUND

As NPs work out their own ideas of what it means to be independent providers, they cannot escape the reality of having to account for physicians. This accounting is not just ideological; it is practical. When NPs and physicians meet in shared terrain, it is usually the NP who carries the weight of making the relationship work. In Stanton's classrooms, nursing faculty would recount personal experiences of having to prove their clinical competence anew whenever they changed jobs or had to work with a new set of physicians. These stories were not narrated as complaints but as a matter-of-fact reality that a collaborating physician might need time to "become comfortable" with an NP's decisions. To be an NP is to shoulder the invisible burden of making these interactions work. In the through-the-looking-glass world of the Grove, the physicians had their own interactional burdens to bear. No one questioned their expertise, but within a nurse-managed organization, there were open questions about their purpose. Given the growing centrality of clinic work, this questioning centered on how they should respond to the Grove's organizational demands.

In this chapter, I explore the ways in which the presence of the NPs is both a cause and a consequence of the changing organization of medical work. While NPs are often thought of as filling in for physicians, at the Grove I observed that there were new pressures on the physicians to fill in for the NPs. In the face of these pressures, the physicians marshaled the traditional prerogative of being a professional and engaged in acts of refusal. These refusals had the intended effect of protecting their status and expertise, but they had the unintended consequence of leaving even more of medicine's traditional realm of responsibility to nursing. The introduction of the NP into the medical encounter raises questions not only about what uniquely constitutes a physician's work but also about what it means to be a medical expert in modern health care.

Accounting for Physician Unease

The Grove was a difficult place to be a physician. In an organization dedicated to showcasing nursing leadership, there seemed to be a carefully constructed silence around the physicians' role. There was the exclusion of physicians' names from team lists posted in the clinic. There was the conspicuous omission of their presence from Stanton's promotional materials. Few people had anything bad to say about the physicians; they simply said nothing at all. These acts of organizational erasure did not go unnoticed by the physicians. As medical director, Dr. Christine Morgan recognized this erasure more clearly than most. "As a female physician," she shared, "you're used to being ignored or looked over. . . . That you're used to. But to be totally and completely ignored? It's unusual and very weird. It's a little off-putting. It really is."

For the physicians who spent time in the clinic, the feeling of being "looked over" or ignored could sometimes seem like an everyday experience. Ten months into her tenure, I asked Dr. Renee Michaels how she was finding the Grove. She confided, "I'm still trying to find my voice. There is such an emphasis on the nurse practitioner—the nurse—that I tiptoed around for a really long time." When Dr. Tracy Polson first started, her understated way of speaking was often literally drowned out during team meetings. The Grove was probably not the most clinically challenging place each had ever worked, but the experience of having to fight to be heard was its own challenge.

In the world outside the Grove, the physician's leadership is unquestioned. There is certainly conflict and jockeying for status between individual physicians; however, as a group, physicians are, as Christine described it, "pretty close to the top of the food chain." The Grove's positioning of the NP as team leader seemed to throw that food chain into disarray. In some ways, the NPs did so by their mere presence. Physicians understand their relationship to RNs. From the very beginning of their training, physicians have to learn to work with bedside nurses. Individual nurses may differ, but as a group, they are a known quantity. Working with NPs is a somewhat different matter. None of the Grove's physicians had much if any previous experience with NPs. Each would have to figure out how to incorporate this different kind of nurse into his or her internal map of how medical work was organized. When Renee was in her first few weeks of acclimating to the Grove, we passed each other in the hallway. I asked her politely how things were going. She smiled and said, "The primary care nurses here are fabulous!" She then hesitated before adding, "I'm still not sure about the NPs. But the nurses are fantastic." Yet the uncertainty raised by the NPs was deeper than where to situate them in the division of labor. The more pressing question seemed to be what the NPs were doing—or not doing—with the physicians.

As the medical director, Christine had already developed an analysis of "the problem with the NPs." In chapter 3, I describe her view that the NPs seemed to be too busy being nurses to act like physicians. Christine's analysis had a second pillar: the NPs did not know when to stop acting like physicians and let the MDs do their jobs. "There are times," she observed, "when [the NPs] should probably consult us more than they do. I don't know if it's just because they're told from the school of nursing that you should be able to do it all and only utilize your physician as a last resort." Christine was not entirely certain what explained the NPs' reticence to call on the physicians. Yet she was sure that a professional directive "to do it all" was at least part of the problem. "I mean, here you have three full-time, intelligent physicians, essentially at your beck and call. Why aren't you using them?"

Christine may have believed that professional pride explained the NPs' habit of not calling on the physicians more often. Yet this explanation did not square with the views of the NPs. From their vantage point in the clinic, the NPs were facing ever-increasing amounts of work. In a little over ten years, the Grove had grown from a small storefront operation to one serving over four hundred members. The NPs felt the full weight of this growth. It was not just the increased numbers; the members themselves had become an expanded site of work.

When the Grove first opened its doors, it was one of only a handful of comprehensive outpatient organizations eligible for enhanced Medicaid reimbursement. But by 2009, there was a fairly robust market of nursing home alternatives. As state and federal payers began to realize the cost savings of community-based care, the increased flow of public dollars spurred the rise of new service providers. Competing organizations began to actively (and sometimes aggressively, according to many of the Grove's staff) solicit the population of frail elderly who were eligible for the Grove. The Grove offered an attractive set of services, but it required members to give up previous providers and to accept center-based care. Older adults with less intensive needs might be inclined to pick a program that offered fewer services but more flexibility. Irrespective of whether this competition was better or worse for patients, the Grove's staff believed it had the effect of increasing the amount of care and management that newly enrolling members required: only those with the highest set of needs—both social and medical— would choose the Grove over other programs.

Stanton may have sometimes been suspected of not wanting quite so many physicians, but the NPs were not the least bit ambivalent about where they stood. As a group, the NPs had been quite vocal in identifying physician absence as an organizational problem. For years, they had collectively voiced wanting more physician time in the clinic. When it looked like their requests were being met, the NPs were welcoming of each new physician hire. As Renee and then Tracy arrived, the NPs waited expectantly for each to get up to speed so they could share the burden of caring for members. They were hopeful when the Grove traded its part-time medical director for a full-time one. The NPs accepted being the primary care provider of record, but from their perspective, there was still plenty of work to go around.

On the surface, there seemed to be a contradiction between physician underutilization and the NPs' stated desire for physician presence. Even Christine described her experience with the NPs as a conundrum. When she first arrived, she described "getting called into" exam rooms all the time. But as her administrative duties grew and she spent less time in the clinic, the requests all but stopped. "I don't know why." She was less physically available, certainly, but, she pointed out, "they have my cell phone"; in theory, they could call at any time. Beneath the surface, however, there was no puzzle. The NPs *did* want to make use of the physicians' expertise, both to support their patients and to support their own professional growth. However, they wanted to incorporate that expertise into the terrain of clinic work. The physicians struggled to recognize this altered terrain as an appropriate place to practice medicine.

Rejection of Interchangeability

The introduction of the NP was predicated on the logic of interchangeability. Certainly, no one expected NPs to replace all forms of physician labor, but their utility was and continues to be measured as a quantum of physician work. Although the Grove was purported to be a model of nursing excellence, it too relied on this logic. Renee explained, "The way that this whole place was set up, and you've probably heard this from a number of people, [voice lowers] is that patients are told that the NPs can do everything the doctors do [voice returns to normal]." For these physicians, however, the logic of interchangeability was not just unbalanced or uncomfortable; it was a mistake. When asked directly, Renee attributed this impossibility to their difference in training. "My training" she explained, "is different in both length and scope. In both *length* and *scope*. I spent two years sitting in the classroom. I mean *two years* sitting in a classroom. And then two years rotating through a bunch of different settings. And then an additional four years rotating through a bunch of different settings, taking book learning and applying it to what's in front of me."

The observation that physicians have more medical training, however, is an argument that nursing has no interest in refuting. In my interviews with Stanton's NP students as well as with the Grove's NPs, an appreciation for this difference was always close to the surface. In various ways, they expressed the sentiment, "I'm not a doctor; I'm a nurse." This was said with some measure of pride: NPs did not have to be like physicians to legitimate their importance to patient care. But even in the midst of such affirmative assertions, there was often a subtle comparison at work. Without my asking, NPs and future NPs alike could not stop themselves from listing the ways in which nursing came up short when compared to medicine. Physicians, they told me, had "all that schooling," had "years of residency training," and had the knowledge to "take [patient problems] down to the atoms!" This comparison was more than just a collection of individual perspectives; it was part of the embodied experience of being a nurse. While most of the public sees the rigors of medical training and practice from a distance, nurses see it up close and in a setting where medicine does its most exalted work: in the acute care hospital. There is little evidence that NPs in general, and the Grove's NPs specifically, believe that their training is the same as physician training.

More to the point, nursing is deeply committed to protecting its own identity. Especially as they fight for practice independence, NPs have little to gain by being viewed as "junior physicians." The boundary between medicine and nursing may be more porous than either side will admit, but for the Grove's NPs, the difference between themselves and the physicians remained self-evident. For the physicians, it was less so. How could physician difference be appreciated if their work was sometimes indistinguishable from that of the NPs? In response to this ambiguity, the Grove's physicians began performing what sociologists term boundary-work. Boundary-work is the rhetorical heightening of group differences as a strategy through which occupations try to expand into new domains, gain or retain a monopoly on authority, or rebuff encroachments on their autonomy (Gieryn 1983). In its legal protestations against NP independence, the AMA is engaging in a classic form of boundary-work. Yet for individual physicians, outright rejection is not always an option. Physician-owners can always choose to circumscribe NP independence or, if their bottom line can sustain it, choose not to hire them at all. However, entrepreneurship is no longer the norm for US physicians. As employees, physicians may find themselves sharing work with NPs whether they want to or not. In contexts without geographic segregation, the boundary between nursing and medicine becomes increasingly difficult to maintain.

At the Grove, the physicians began to defend their boundaries by enacting both material and symbolic forms of work segregation. Although initially tip-toeing around the NPs, Renee eventually became more assertive in declaring the primacy of the physician's expertise. "There's a certain amount of arrogance on the part of the physician," she said. "Yes, there is. The thing is that there's a certain need, at least on my part, to change the expectation. I'm really good at what I do, so please don't throw the sore toe at me because you don't have time." I initially found her statement curious. "Sore toes" may not be the most exciting of physician concerns, but they—along with runny noses and stomach aches—are squarely on the list of problems to which primary care physicians attend. Throughout the country, other organizations similar to the Grove have clinics staffed primarily by physicians. One assumes those physicians treat sore toes as well as heart failure. However, Renee's evocation of the sore toe was instructive. In a world without NPs, such concerns might still be medical work. But in a world with NPs, something had changed. The wall between medicine and nursing had begun to crumble. Action needed to be taken to restore things to right.

Disavowal of NP Work

As individuals and as a group, the physicians at the Grove began engaging in acts of refusal to do NP work. The most public and consequential act of refusal happened during a moment of acute organizational vulnerability. NP Anne was on vacation, and so was Christine. This put Renee in a stressful position. Under the Grove's default policy, Renee would be expected to fill in for the missing NP. But she was also asked to take on some of the medical director's clinical responsibilities. It was a perfect storm that revealed the cracks in several of the Grove's organizational logics.

One of these was the logic of provider interchangeability. Renee described her breaking point in this way: "I was trying to do my job and covering for Anne as best I could. And covering for part of Christine's job. And then I was asked to do something else, and I said no." Renee did not say no behind closed doors; she said it during morning meeting. One of the various lists read each morning contained the names of new members. The purpose was to alert the team to prioritize their enrollment assessments. On this morning, Anne's team had a new enrollment. In her absence, someone else had to do the medical assessment. Based on the logic of interchangeability, Renee was asked to fill in and complete it.

Each assessment took the NPs approximately an hour for the visit, followed by a comprehensive entry in the medical record that took thirty minutes to an hour to complete.[1] Given the weight of the work, it was not surprising that this was the task that shattered the illusion of NP-physician interchangeability. From Renee's perspective, she was asked to do "something else." But this "something else" was a standard part of the NPs' work in the clinic. At this fateful morning meeting, Renee stood up and said—calmly but not completely without emotion—that she did not have the time. Moreover, she should not be asked to cover for Anne. "The NPs," she said firmly, "should cover for each other."

Her suggested fix required that a new organizational distinction be made between NP work and physician work. Renee would later observe that not everyone was supportive of her taking a stand. She attributed this lack of support to an organizational culture of not saying no. I had a slightly different reading of the situation. Renee did not simply say no. Her public complaint did not include being asked to take on the medical director's work. She said no specifically to taking on the work of the NPs. She was rejecting the logic of interchangeability and refusing to be made over into a nurse.

Renee's rejection not only revealed cracks in the logic of interchangeability but also shattered another illusion—that the NPs and the physicians were on the same team. The team was no longer an entity whose members pitched in for one another, but rather, NPs helped NPs; physicians helped physicians. Such a vision had already been tested in smaller, less public ways. As I describe in chapter 3, individual physicians failed to do NP work almost any time an NP was away from the clinic.

These individual acts of refusal notwithstanding, Renee's public refusal laid bare what lay behind physician resistance. It was not about "sore toes" or workplace efficiency; it was a refusal to accept the proposition that NPs and physicians could or should do the same work. Renee's complaint became part of a broader boundary-work campaign to reassert physician difference. Renee believed her refusal "wasn't taken well." That may have been true from an interpersonal standpoint, but in other ways, it went about as well as it could have. Her public refusal became the catalyst for organizational change. Not long after, the medical director and director of nursing announced a new policy. The NPs would now be formally expected to cover for one another. The physicians no longer had to refuse to do the work of NPs as individuals. They were exempted as a distinct category of provider.

Renee had herself used the word "arrogance" to account for physician resistance to doing NP work. Certainly, inhabiting the top of any hierarchy requires a certain amount of confidence. However, I am not persuaded that the behavior of the physicians was motivated by mere ego. None of these physicians had been drafted to work at the Grove. Each one had willingly signed on to work for an organization that not only emphasized nursing practice but also featured the

NP as the primary care provider. As Renee put it, "I think it takes a very specific kind of individual to want to do geriatric medicine. And then to want to do it in a structure that is meant to be nurse practitioner driven? It may not be the way most people want to do things." But the physicians at the Grove were each the "kind of individual" willing to do so. The Grove's nursing identity may not have been its chief attraction, but neither was it a hurdle to taking the job. Yet in spite of this willingness, the reality of working at the Grove was unsettling in a way that went beyond bruised pride. For the physicians, a clinic inhabited by NPs was no longer an appropriate place for medicine. In this context, the problem seemed to be less that the NPs thought they were physicians, than that the physicians began to feel as if they were becoming NPs.

The threat to the physicians was not just in being pressed to do NP work, but also in being asked to support NP-defined understandings of what kind of work was needed. When NP Stephen stepped into his role as the director of nursing, he stepped into the unresolved question of what it was the physicians should be doing. When I spoke with him about this question, he began by defining the NPs' role. "Any conference I go to, they always cite the seventy-thirty rule: 70 percent of what a person presents to you in a primary care office should be able to be handled by an NP. . . . Well, that means that about 30 percent of the time you should be on the phone with one of your physicians, saying, 'I need your brain.'" He contrasted this approach with the complaints that came from the physicians: that the NPs would summarily hand them work, saying, "I ran out of time so could you go see these three people."

I never witnessed this exact conversation between an NP and physician. But I did hear a similar concern from Renee. Ten months into her tenure, she began to get frustrated by the NPs' growing impatience. "They've been asking me for a schedule—'when are you available to us'—since I started." One could interpret this impatience as NP appreciation for what the physicians had to offer. But Renee did not feel appreciated; she felt disrespected. Her summation of NP expectations were, "We need you to be sitting in the clinic because when I get overwhelmed, I need to be able to just start pushing people your way." Still, I did not fully understand Renee's perspective until I observed what happened, not between a physician and an NP, but between a physician and a primary care nurse.

When NP Norah was away on vacation, one of the things I noticed was the new work that Joanne, her primary care nurse, took on in her absence. It was easier to recognize it as work when it was not quietly done as an everyday routine but grappled with as something slightly unfamiliar. One of those forms of work was the management of the physician's schedule. I already knew that Norah made Tracy's schedule. If Norah wanted to get her members seen, she took responsibility for getting them in front of the physician. But what I had not realized was how much active management this required. One morning, I watched Joanne make Tracy's schedule. She first looked over the list of members who needed to be seen in clinic and compared it with the list of who was in the center. When Joanne saw Tracy in the hall that morning, she called out loudly and with an uncharacteristic, forced cheerfulness, "Mr. Jacobs is in the center today. He has been on your list forever! So you can see him. Okay?" Tracy answered, "Okay," with neither a smile nor any evidence of enthusiasm. Later that afternoon, Joanne had been reading an email exchange about a member. She determined he needed to be seen. She called the front desk and said, "Please add Mr. Peter Thompson to Dr. Polson's schedule." Noticeably, she did not call Tracy to let her know.

Throughout Norah's absence, Joanne made decisions about what Tracy needed to do. Whether a visit needed to happen on a given day was not simply a matter of medical acuity or whether only the physician's expertise would do; it was a balancing act of knowing how often a member came in, and whether the visit was generated by an administrative need or a member need. These were all calculations that Norah would normally make and that Joanne was making in her stead, but none of these calculations was made in consultation with the physicians. All the physicians knew was that a group of nurses seemed to be constantly telling them what to do and how to do it.

As the frontline clinician for member care, it was the NP, or her primary care nurse proxy, who decided when problems should be brought to a physician's attention. Moreover, placed in charge of managing clinic work, the NPs often were in a position to dictate how that work should be done. As a consequence, physician work was in danger of being defined more by NPs' needs than by those of patients. Christine's statement that the physicians were at the NPs' "beck and call" was probably intended more for dramatic effect than as sober description. But for the physicians who worked in the clinic, it was a rather prescient warning of what could happen if they were not vigilant. In the Grove's clinic, there was still work that only physicians could do, but that work was increasingly being defined by nursing's prerogatives rather than those of medicine.

I began to understand that the source of the physicians' unease was less about their exclusion and more about the terms of their inclusion. In the world outside the Grove, the physician remains the normative ideal. An NP might be mistaken for a physician, but to mistake a lower-status professional for one with higher status is an error rather than an affront. In some quarters, it might even be considered a compliment. At the Grove, the error was more likely to go the other way. No one literally mistook the physicians for NPs. But with the NPs acting as the default providers, the physicians were in danger of being pressed into performing and supporting the NP-defined domain of clinic work. In this setting, the blur-ring of professional boundaries served less to elevate the NPs than to demote the physicians.

Denial of NP Authority

At the Grove, the status of the physicians was threatened, not by rejection, but by the ways in which the NPs tried to include them. The notion that the current physicians' jobs were defined by when and how the NPs needed them echoed the complaints of the previous group of physicians. Renee described the NPs as wanting "to be able to email you and have you stand up from your desk and come in and attend to what [they are] attending to right now. That's happened a number of times." No one, however, goes to medical school to be given orders; one goes to medical school to give them.

"In all of the careers in health care I've looked at, the physician gets to be in charge. I don't want somebody else telling me what to do." This was the answer a younger Renee gave when an interviewer for a postbaccalaureate program asked her, "Why become a physician and not a nurse?" Perhaps this was a standard interview question, but it may have been directed at Renee specifically. At the time of her application to the program, Renee was already thirty-seven years old. She was married and the mother of a young son. This is not the typical profile of an aspiring physician. Despite the rise of alternative pathways to medicine, medical school remains the province of the young. In 2017, the mean age of US medical school matriculants was twenty-four (Association of American Medical Colleges 2017). While other professions attract late-career entrants, medicine has a hurdle that is difficult to overcome in later life: time.

Medical training in the US is fairly unique in the length of its commitment. Medical school applicants have already completed a four-year bachelor's degree. After that, prospective physicians face an additional seven to fourteen years of schooling. Typically, four years of medical school are followed by at least three years of residency for primary care specialties and up to seven for rarified fields such as neurosurgery. For some specialties, a post-residency fellowship of one to three years is expected. The weight of this time commitment is measured not just in years but in hours. In 2003, the Accreditation Council for Graduate Medical Education instituted new regulations that lowered the workweek of residents to a still quite formidable 80 hours, although surveys of residents suggest that many feel both internal and external pressures to keep to the pre-2003 norm of 120 hours (Drolett et al. 2013; Landrigan et al. 2006).

Whether a resident's work week is 80 hours, 120 hours, or something in between, this kind of time requirement is often an insurmountable hurdle for the not-so-young adult with preexisting commitments. In the face of these challenges, many people in Renee's situation choose differently. Stephen was almost exactly the same age as Renee when he chose nursing. He told me that he had long ago considered a career in medicine, but as a college student, he was not ready for the long and narrow road that led to medicine. "I just wanted to be a more renaissance-type person." Stephen went on to build a successful career in the corporate world, but he began to feel like there was something else he should be doing. "I was getting close to forty, and I just couldn't shake it. I couldn't shake that desire. City University kept advertising for this accelerated BSN. So one day I just applied. I just said that's it. I'm done."

I asked Stephen why he chose nursing rather than his original dream of medicine. His response was succinct: "Age." I was surprised by this answer, given his vocal desire to champion the nursing profession. When I asked him to elaborate on this seeming contradiction, he was frank. "Look," he said. "I'm not immune to the pressures of society. And there's a lot of prestige about being a doctor. I mean, the public loves nurses, but they'll genuflect to a doctor." If Stephen had been a younger man with the chance to do it over again, there was no question that he would have become a doctor. "Medicine," he said, "is still where the power is." For both Renee and Stephen, health care was a domain in which the physician remained the one in charge. It is not only the rigors of medical training but also the personal sacrifices it requires that legitimate that position.

Those sacrifices were not inconsequential. For Renee, a desire for status alone would not have been enough to sustain her through the journey ahead. Medicine seemed like something she had spent her whole life talking herself out of. She had already tried several "good enough" careers. But medicine was beginning to feel like something she was called to do. One summer, she decided to "dip her toe in the water" through a summer volunteer program at a local hospital. "By the time the program was done, that was it. I was hooked."

For Renee, the way forward was clear but far from simple. She had to bypass the doubts of others, like the interviewer who asked why she wanted to pursue medicine and not nursing. She had to get into and complete a postbaccalaureate program just to be eligible to apply to medical school. Then there was the training. Renee was, on average, sixteen years older than most of her classmates. She recalled her amazement over how much faster her younger colleagues seemed to learn the material. But Renee also had the additional work of keeping her family together throughout her training. "That I got to keep my child and husband in a relatively normal relationship throughout the whole process is amazing to me.... I guess my husband and I really wanted this relationship to work." It was also clear that she wanted medicine to work. She stuck with it through medical school, residency, and a one-year geriatric fellowship.

Renee had initially chosen medicine so she could be the one in charge. The intervening years had not exactly changed her mind, but they had leavened her perspective. The AMA, with its sometimes singular focus on protecting physician power, is not the only voice of the profession. Some would argue that it is not even the most representative voice. In 2016, only 25 percent of practicing physicians held AMA membership (American Medical Association 2017). There are many physicians who champion the values of teamwork and collaboration. These alternative voices have influenced both medical education and professional norms.

Renee was a product of these new influences. When she was the not-quite-so-new physician at the Grove, I asked how she was finding the position. Although the conversation would eventually wind its way to the challenges, it was telling that she began with a declaration of affection: "I love working as part of a team. I love it!" This affection was not a new feeling; she located its beginnings in medical school. Studying for tests together was something she found so gratifying that she didn't want it to stop there. "I wanted to take the test together, and I wanted to, you know, practice together." That love of team-based practice was cemented when she finished her training. One of the first positions she held was as a medical director for an inpatient hospice program. At hospice, she worked with social workers, nurses, aides, and chaplains. "I love the idea that we're working together with all of our different skills and trainings."

Given her previous background, the Grove's model of team-based care was not a radical departure. Moreover, she, as well as the other physicians, voiced unanimous support for the idea that everyone on the team had a distinct and important role to play in patient care. But because NPs and physicians addressed similar problems, it was a challenge for the physicians to accept NP expertise without modifying their understanding of their own. To resolve this dilemma, the physicians continued their boundary-work campaign by denying the possibility of NP authority.

In chapter 4, I show that the physicians dealt with their uneasiness with the NP role by discursively incorporating the NP as a subordinate. NP Francesca, the scribe who had offered me the Venn diagram, voiced her dissatisfaction with this understanding of nursing. She noted, "While we have respect for what's over here in medicine, [the physicians] have no respect for this whole chunk of things called nursing because medical decisions always trump nursing decisions." When I asked for an example, she described a case in which one of the previous physicians had vetoed her recommendation for inpatient rehabilitation after a surgery but she, based on her knowledge of the patient's resources, knew the member would not be able to manage self-care at home. The physician ended the conversation with the assessment that rehab "was not medically necessary." Francesca, however, felt he had missed the point; it may not have been medically necessary, but it was necessary if one considered the whole person. I do not doubt the veracity of Francesca's story, but it was not apparent from my own observations that this was a common problem. What she described as the trumping of nursing decisions often seemed less about what the physicians demanded and more about the NPs' willingness to acquiescence to medical authority. But sometimes the logic that undergirds a situation is most clearly seen in aberrant rather than in normal encounters.

I observed such an encounter during one of Norah's team meetings. As the team's physician, Tracy was in attendance along with everyone else. She was still in her first six months at the Grove and had not quite gotten her bearings in terms of how things worked. However, she did not let this bother her. She had been a practicing physician for well over thirty years. Although reserved, she was well accustomed to the mantle of authority required of her profession. It did not take long for that authority to be tested.

Norah seemed to run her team meetings by the strength of her personality. Unlike some other teams, there was no standardized agenda; there was no formal facilitator. Norah's conversational style often made it difficult to even know exactly when the meeting had shifted from premeeting chatter to substantive conversation. Yet every week, her team covered what needed to be covered and decided what needed to be decided. As I attended these meetings week after week, I began to see how Norah kept the meeting going in the right direction with a rhythm of open-floor storytelling followed by decisive decision-making about next steps. She had a way of weaving everyone's stories into a singular narrative of which she was the primary author.

When Tracy first began attending these meetings, her voice was rarely heard. Norah never directly asked for her input. The structure and rhythm that Norah had established seemed to leave little space for distinctly medical problems. However, in one meeting, a discrete medical issue presented itself. Norah had just finished summarizing the clinical notes pertaining to Ms. Howard's six-month assessment. As part of that assessment, Norah had run through Ms. Howard's long list of medical problems, concluding that most of them were being stably managed, with the notable exception of lower-extremity edema, or swelling in her legs. While she had more than one medical condition that contributed to this problem, its chronic nature was exacerbated by the barriers she faced in elevating her legs at night. Like many members with physical limitations, Ms. Howard preferred to spend her evenings and nights in a reclining chair in her living room rather than to struggle to get into bed. With her legs always in a dependent position, swelling was destined to remain an intractable problem.

After listening to this assessment, Tracy recommended that Norah try taking Ms. Howard off Gabapentin, a nonopioid medication that she took for chronic pain. Tracy's reasoning was that one of the side effects of Gabapentin was lower-extremity edema. In an unusual reaction, Norah resisted. "You don't know long it took me to get her pain under control." For Norah, the complication was that Ms. Howard was a former abuser of controlled substances. Finding a nonopioid medication that adequately addressed her pain had created stability in her treatment regime, which Norah described as previously being quite tumultuous. Tracy quietly stood her ground, refusing to cede the point. In the face of physician authority, Norah acquiesced and moved the discussion on to the next member case.

I stopped by Norah's office later that afternoon. She filled in more about the situation of Ms. Howard. "I remember when she was stealing [a family member's] pain medication." She had become a frequent flyer in the clinic, coming into Norah's office every day, tearfully complaining of pain. A tearful and narcotic-stealing Ms. Howard was both a medical problem and an organizational problem. It was not just Ms. Howard who would come in every day with complaints; Norah would be confronted with a cascade of complaints from Ms. Howard's home care nurses and aides. For Norah, finding an effective pain medication was not just a matter of balancing the benefits and side effects of a medical intervention; it was also about managing the totality of Ms. Howard's problems. Norah's countering of Tracy's assessment was based on a questioning not of her medical knowledge but of her knowledge of the patient. However, this knowledge was patently dismissed by the physician. It was not simply that Tracy did not yield; there was no room for negotiation. As mild as it was, such open, public disagreement between an NP and a physician was almost singular in its rarity. However, it was through this rare event that one could see the normal state of affairs more clearly. The recognition of expertise between physician and NP was not mutual. The physicians did not accept the possibility of a separate well of NP expertise. As a consequence, the idea that an NP might be able to speak authoritatively about a patient was inconceivable.

The denial of NP authority was illustrated more explicitly in another part of the organization when there was the possibility that a nurse might claim more expertise over an area of medical knowledge. That was the situation that NP Bridgette found herself in. Bridgette had a unique position at the Grove. Her formal title was "clinical educator." She was a geriatric NP, but she had also earned a PhD in nursing research. Stanton had hired her because of her expertise in clinical research and geriatric practice. While there was still some question regarding how the Grove would use that expertise, she had settled into a role as a geriatric psychiatric consultant. This put her in an interesting position: By whom would she be considered an expert? Which providers would she be allowed to educate?

Bridgette came to the Grove not just with a wealth of clinical experience but with a lot of previous experience collaborating with physicians. "I am so used to problem-solving with a physician and not just pulling them in when I can't figure it out. In nursing home practice, I would round with the physician and bring up issues I was concerned about or had a suspicion about. . . . It's nice to be able to communicate and kind of think through whether the pieces you're putting together make sense." She did not need to be in charge, but she was accustomed to having her expertise acknowledged. In addition to positive experiences collaborating with physicians, she had trained medical residents and geriatric fellows because she had "the twenty-five years of experience and the knowledge base to do that." However, her transition to the Grove was not easy. "It's a nurse-run organization and it should, at the very least, be equal. But there's just some weird dynamics that go on and I don't get it." She continued, "I really had a Rodney Dangerfield experience where you just—like Dr. Morgan had no idea that my title was doctor. Two years into this position and she didn't really know that, and I'm like, how did she not know that?"

Bridgette recounted one of these "Rodney Dangerfield" moments when she tried to put her twenty-five years of experience to use at an organizational level. She had developed a standardized template for the NPs and physicians to use on their nursing home visits. She described getting feedback from the providers at a primary care meeting and had eventually gotten approval by the medical director. Later, she found the template had not been implemented. When she asked Christine about it, she was told, "We decided that the nurse practitioners wouldn't do the nursing home visits anymore so we didn't need that." Bridgette recalls, "I just looked right at her and said, 'I did not make that note just for the nurse practitioners. I made that note for the physicians [too]. They're missing significant geriatric syndromes on their visits.' I said, 'That is why I developed that template. . . . I shouldn't be finding on [my own] gero-psych visits a fifteen-pound weight loss, having been seen by the physician three times and they never noticed that the patient had lost fifteen pounds. Or that the patient has a wound and the physician hasn't documented it, or that they're depressed and the physician hasn't clued in to that, or you know, poly pharmacy.' I just went through all these geriatric syndromes, and she said, 'Well, I don't like check-offs. We're not going to use it.'" According to Bridgette, they did not argue science or the evidence; there was no conversation at all. Bridgette could be an expert for the NPs but not for the physicians. This refusal to recognize nursing expertise was related to the physicians' reworking of the medical hierarchy to include the NPs only as skilled subordinates. This reworking held all physicians above all nurses, regardless of individual experience or knowledge.

This reassertion of physicians as a superordinate class of provider distinct from and above the NPs was also enacted at the organizational level. One place it could be seen was through organizational meetings. Primary care meetings happened every Friday at midday. While the agenda changed over time, the guiding principle was evaluating and improving the work that occurred in the clinic. How well were the teams completing their six-month assessments? What were the problems with documentation in the electronic medical record? How might they fix problems with clinic flow? While the agenda changed and shifted over time, I began to notice a systematic pattern—not of what was included, but of what was excluded. These meetings were never the site of discussions about how the physicians managed or organized their work. Such discussions happened in a separate meeting where only the physicians were present. Because the NPs were stationed in the clinic, clinic problems were synonymous with NP problems. The work of the NPs was up for global critique; physician work was talked about only among physicians.

The one-way nature of this dynamic was difficult to see because it seemed perfectly reasonable for the physicians to meet separately to discuss matters that affected only them. However, there were times when the opaqueness of physician decisions was not just a practical matter but a symbolic assertion of power. One of those occasions was in how the newly changed leave policy worked when the physician was away. Tracy was forced to take an extended medical leave of absence. Just as the NPs were expected to make their own plan when one of their own was out, the physicians took the same responsibility to do so. However, what was telling was less the plan itself than how it was communicated.

"This is what's going to happen and here's how you're going to do it." This was how Francesca described the email the NPs received from Christine. Francesca contrasted this episode to what happened when Michelle had been out on medical leave. "All the NPs and physicians sat at the table and said, 'Michelle will be out this long. How can we manage the work load?' And we divided it up and came up with your plan. This time Tracy will be out and you get *this* from the medical director. I know I'm ultrasensitive to this but 'Dr. Morgan' and 'Dr. Michaels' at the bottom? It just doesn't feel good. There's been a lot of bitching about that email." The email was sent from the medical director's account, but it was signed by the physicians as a group: "Dr. Morgan and Dr. Michaels." The physicians had not just become a separate group of providers; they were speaking with one voice as an administrative category over the NPs. Supervision may not have been the dominant model in use at the Grove, but the physicians were not reticent to evoke it in order to repair the boundary between themselves and the NPs.

In chapter 4, I describe how the physicians engaged in material acts of work segregation by moving more of their work outside the clinic. Here, I have illustrated the symbolic ways in which they asserted their difference from and superordinate status to the NPs. In many ways, these strategies were successful. In refusing to do NP work, recognize NP authority, or even, at times, be found in the same location as NPs, they were able to repair the breach. Anyone who mistook them for NPs or expected them to take on clinic work eventually found themselves corrected. Yet, as successful as the physicians may have been in preserving their status, these strategies were also, in their own way, acts of capitulation. When patients and staff went to the clinic, it was the NPs they found there, not the physicians. The physicians' status may have been protected, but they had ceded a certain amount of ground to do so.

Organizational Gains, Physician Losses

Professional medicine has been remarkably successful in protecting its status and expertise. However, an exclusive focus on what the profession has won has perhaps obscured what individual physicians have lost. At the Grove and in much of health care, physicians are being pushed out of the clinic as much as they can be said to have affirmatively left. At the Grove, the physicians found themselves in an altered medical landscape, facing a new set of constraints. To stay meant to practice in a fundamentally different way with a changed set of relationships, not only with NPs but also with their employer. There remained a small but shrinking place for their expertise, but there was seemingly no place left for them. Leaving the clinic was an act of capitulation, but it was not to nursing; it was to the rising power of health care organizations.

This is a story that has been played out in health care for at least three decades. It is a story that is illustrated in the career biographies of physicians like Christine. Before becoming the Grove's medical director, Christine had spent her entire career in primary care. Just a few years after completing her residency in internal medicine, Christine was hired by a physician-owned practice: Newton Medical Services. Newton Medical was a community-based internal medicine practice. Nestled within the same neighborhoods that the Grove would eventually serve, Newton Medical was the equivalent of "a small-town doc" for local residents. Christine and her colleagues saw adults of every age, for every condition, at every stage of life. She would stay at Newton for almost seventeen years. While some of her patients would come and go, she developed ongoing, meaningful relationships with others. When I asked her why she left the practice where she had invested so much of her life, she told a story that was partly personal but also reflected larger shifts in US medicine. Christine may have stayed at the same workplace, but the work had changed around her in ways that made moving on seem like the right thing to do.

When Christine entered the medical workforce, physician-owned practices were the predominant organizational form for primary care. It was not surprising that she found herself working in such a setting. She worked alongside three other internists, two of whom owned the practice. Reminiscing about those early days, Christine recalled, "We had such a good time." Although she was an employee, she was working with the owners as much as for them. It was also an opportunity to practice the kind of medicine she had grown to love in residency. "There really wasn't anything that I liked or found intellectually or scientifically stimulating outside of internal medicine." An internist has "to know a little bit about a whole lot of different things" in order to manage the complexity of a patient's entire medical profile. Some medical students reject primary care specialties because of the unchanging parade of diabetes, hypertension, and heart disease; physicians like Christine find the individual variation fascinating. "Even if I spend the day seeing ten people with diabetes, everybody's diabetes is different. It's still all diabetes but it's all different. . . . That's something that sort of came to me the more I got to do and see more medicine."

She could not have known it then, but those good times were about to end. In 1995, Stanton University Hospital approached Newton Medical's owners to see whether they wanted to sell. They declined. But when they were approached again, a year later, they said yes. Christine did not know why they changed their minds. As an employee of the practice, she was "not really privy to the inner workings." But she did not need any secret knowledge to see what was happening in front of her eyes. The traditional model of physician entrepreneurship was under assault.

Hospitals around the country were buying up private practices at a rapidly increasing pace (Goldsmith 1993). Hospitals were not really interested in the relatively unprofitable primary care market. Their strategy was to leverage practice ownership to secure patient referrals and hospital admissions. Then and now, most patients rely on their primary care providers for referrals for specialists; for expensive diagnostic tests such as x-rays, CT scans, and colonoscopies; for recommendations on where to go for surgical procedures; and even suggestions for which hospital's emergency department they should go to. If hospitals could increase their market share of primary care practices, they would be able to increase their market share of more lucrative hospital-based services. The economic logic seemed sound; however, hospitals found themselves competing with each other for a finite resource. Many hospitals got caught up in open bidding wars, offering owners what in hindsight were highly inflated prices (O'Malley, Bond, and Berenson 2011). Physician-owners were often the winners in these transactions; many made a tidy profit at the expense of hospitals, but these were not unmitigated wins. The hospitals were economic Goliaths; many physicians feared being driven out of business if they held out too long. As a consequence of increased competition from hospital-owned practices, many independent owners felt pressured into selling.

Whatever the reasons were for Newton Medical's decision to sell, in 1996, Christine found herself an employee of Stanton Health System. Stanton merged Newton with a nearby practice, acquiring both new patients and new providers. According to Christine, concerns with profitability began to lean more heavily on the doors of the exam room. Newton Medical had always been a business, but suddenly "there were all sorts of pressures from the hierarchy to try and see more people; to make more money." Stanton also added nursing home residents to Newton's panel of patients. Christine began traveling to nursing homes throughout the city in addition to seeing patients in the office.

Few physicians practice medicine as a nine-to-five proposition, but Christine's days began to seem endless. She recalled spending eleven to twelve hours a day at work, just trying to keep her head above water. "I would round in the hospital, be in the office, and then go to the nursing home towards the end of the day. It was exhausting." If she "made it home early," she would arrive by seven with just enough time to kiss her children on their way to bed. In the quiet of the evening, she would then begin her second shift, sorting through the "volumes and volumes and volumes of paper" she brought home each night. "Every test that you ordered, every lab that you had, every consult that you sent somebody to generated paper" that had to be reviewed. "Being in private practice is tough. It's very tough."

There was, however, a small glimmer of silver in these increasingly long days. "As time moved on and . . . my patients were aging, I found that I was really sort of more drawn to the geriatric portion of my patient base than the younger folks." Her visits to the nursing home, although initially just another burden, became the best part of her day. "I found that when I was in the nursing home, my blood pressure was lower than if I took it at the end of the day in the office. Somewhere along the way, the light bulb went on: maybe I need to just get out of the office." She began spending as little time in the office as she could and devoted more and more of her time to the nursing home. She recalled, "I wasn't happy," but she had found a way to hang on. And practically speaking, she did not have the time or energy to actively look for another job. Taking refuge in the nursing home was an imperfect solution, but it was good enough. Until it wasn't.

Stanton Health System soon began considering yet another revenue-generating policy for the practice: evening clinic hours. For Christine, this was a clarifying moment. "That was *not* on my list of things to do. To stay down here until nine o'clock? No!" While she had been mulling over what she wanted to do in her working life, her life at home had already moved on to a different phase. Married Christine had become divorced Christine. As a self-described "single mom," the prospect of evening clinic hours was not just unpalatable but untenable. Something would have to change. That change would appear in the form of an email that inquired, "Would you be interested in this?"

The email was from the Grove's outgoing medical director. He had been with the Grove from the beginning. But as a part-time administrator, he felt he could not meet the needs of the growing organization. He was convinced that the Grove needed a dedicated, full-time medical director; he was also convinced that this was not something he wanted to take on. Leading the search for his own replacement, he reached out to Christine. As she read the job description, she remembered thinking, "This could solve all my problems." After years in the trenches, an administrative position might provide some relief from the never-ending grind of private practice. The Grove's exclusive focus on older adults would transform her clinical side gig into the main event. For Christine, the email was "like an omen."

But omens portend losses as well as gains. Christine had not fully considered the prospect of leaving her patients behind. "I had seen [my patients] for so long that I became part of their family—which is something they never tell you in medical school. It's something that I wasn't even prepared for." She decided to send in her resume; but even then, she hoped she could figure out a way to keep one foot in private practice. Perhaps she could persuade the Grove to accept a highly motivated part-time medical director. By her calculations, even a part-time administrative position might buy her out of the most unpleasant parts of private practice while enabling her to keep her longtime patients. But during her first interview, those hopes began to fall away. The more she learned about the Grove, the more she realized how much their vision required "somebody to be here, 100 percent of the time."

When Christine was invited back for a second interview, the reality of what she was doing could no longer be ignored. "I really had to think long and hard and talk to various people." One person she sought counsel from was her mother. Her mother's first words were ones of shock. "You can't give up your practice! How are you going to walk out?" These words amplified Christine's own doubts: How could she? How could she just pack up and leave? "I know," she answered, to herself as much as to her mother. "But it's killing me."

The more she thought about it, the more it began to seem that the position at the Grove was its own calling, of sorts. "I kept thinking, 'It just popped into my inbox.' You know? This is probably something that I'm supposed to do." But she also accepted that she would be giving something up in the bargain. Christine would still practice medicine. She would still see patients and consult on their care. But she would not be anyone's doctor in quite the same way again. It was the end of an era for Christine. But it had long been the end of an era for medicine.

Nurse practitioners might be seen as simply the latest iteration of contests over jurisdiction between two perennially dueling groups (Abbott 1988). If the Grove is any indication, nursing may gain new concessions from each new skirmish, but the physicians will ultimately win. At the Grove, physicians remained at the top of the medical hierarchy, even in the aberrant terrain of a nurse-managed organization. Their position of leadership was not just symbolic; they were able to wield their authority in ways that mattered for NP practice. The physicians could participate in acts of refusal that the NPs would have found impossible. In the aftermath of Renee's refusal to do the work of an NP, one NP wondered aloud, "Can you imagine what would have happened if I stood up in morning meeting and just refused to do something?" I cannot imagine what would have happened, primarily because I cannot imagine that an NP at the Grove would have done so. I am also reminded that the rather mild refusals that Michelle engaged in were officially censured.

The contests at the Grove, however, were not just between medicine and nurses; they were also about the changing relationship between bureaucratic health care organizations and the providers they employ. There are distinct pressures on what it means to be a physician in the modern health care organization. As seen through Christine's career narrative, the prerequisites of being a professional have never only been about status. For individual providers, being a professional is also about the conditions of work. For physicians, this has meant, to some degree, a guarantee of protection: from patients at times, but mostly from the demands of organizations and, by extension, those of payers. A hospital might seek the expertise of a physician, but physicians have historically provided such services as independent consultants. Hospital managers can and have structured the work of clerks, custodians, aides, and nurses, but how long a surgery lasts, what medications are dispensed, and which clinical interventions are implemented—these matters are largely up to the physician. This protection is usually touted as a way to secure patient access to evidenced-based care, but it is equally a protection of the physician's working conditions.

Nurse practitioners are the heirs of both nursing's different view of patients and nursing's different relationship to employers; as a consequence, NPs are much more pliant providers than physicians. The obligation that nursing enacts toward an expansive set of problems is not just about a gendered notion of care work; it is also about a different relationship with employers. The Grove's NPs were called to be women of the organization as well as women of the profession. The physicians' rejection of clinic work was a rejection of a changed relationship with their employer as much as with nursing. These physicians still had enough cultural and political power to resist change; however, their primary mode of resistance was through abdication, leaving the NPs to meet the medical needs of their shared patients, alone.

Part III

A SHRINKING TERRAIN FOR SOCIAL PROBLEMS

THE CONTRACTION OF SOCIAL WORK

It was Friday morning, and we had all just sat through NP Norah's team meeting. As Norah was gathering up her pile of papers, she turned to social worker (SW) Margaret and said, seemingly out of the blue, "Mr. Harvey met his son." Margaret's eyes opened wide. "Oh really?" For Norah, that was enough of an invitation to begin telling the kind of long and descriptive story that distinguished her as the expert of her members.

Mr. Harvey had enrolled in the Grove as a widower. Before that, he had been living with his wife and a disabled grandson. When his wife became ill, Mr. Harvey took out loans and mortgaged his house to help pay for her care. "By the time she died," Norah explained, "he was penniless." When Mr. Harvey could not make the mortgage payment, the house went into foreclosure. He and his grandson faced homelessness. The story of a homeless widower and his disabled grandson made the Channel 6 news. According to Norah, one of the people who felt moved by the news feature was Mr. Harvey's niece. She called the news station and put herself forward as someone who wanted to help. Part of what had moved her was not just the plight of Mr. Harvey, but that of his grandson. "Because it turns out," noted Norah, "she was already raising the grandson's half-sister, who is also disabled." The niece originally volunteered to take in just the grandson, but when she saw how close they were, she took in Mr. Harvey as well.

Mr. Harvey had found a stable home with people who made sure he was taken care of. In managing his care and providing day care services, the Grove played a key part in helping Mr. Harvey's niece support him. However, Mr. Harvey's progressive dementia threatened to disrupt the carefully orchestrated threads of his life. Mr. Harvey needed surgery, and there was no one with the legal authority to give the surgeon permission to proceed. Mr. Harvey was not competent enough to make the decision himself. His niece was comfortable providing for Mr. Harvey through the bonds of family and affection, but not the bonds of legality. She was not willing to make medical decisions on his behalf. Without a close family member or a designated power of attorney, the surgeon was reluctant to proceed outside of a life-threatening emergency.

Norah did what she often did when faced with a hurdle standing between a member and medical care. Fixing the problem was not just something she felt compelled do, but something she considered to be her job. She did her own sleuthing and "dug up a son" from a previous marriage. He and Mr. Harvey hadn't spoken in over five years. But Norah arranged a meeting. "He was surprised at how old his father looked. He kept saying, 'Your hair is white!'" It was a heartwarming story to be sure. But Norah had not done this sleuthing for the purposes of family reunification. For Norah, this was a case of medical necessity. The son marveled at his father's appearance; he also gave his consent for the surgery to proceed.

As I listened to this account, it struck me that this could have been Margaret's story instead of Norah's. It could have been the story of how the social worker's attention to family dynamics and relationships helped to facilitate access to health care. Yet at the Grove, these kinds of stories were reflective of the work that happened in the clinic, rather than through social work. This was only one of many cases in which the Grove's social workers did not seem to be doing the kind of work I imagined they might do. In fact, they did not seem to be doing the kind of work that even they imagined belonged to them.

When I asked the social workers to describe their role on the team, their answers hewed fairly closely to the following: coordinating care, connecting members and families with resources, and helping to solve "sticky" problems that threatened to get in the way of member well-being. Given this description, the case of Mr. Harvey would seem to have fit squarely in social work's domain. Yet this problem, and many others like it, did not make it onto the social workers' to-do lists. Instead, they made it onto the NPs'. If the NPs were doing this kind of work from inside the clinic, what were the social workers doing outside it? As I observed how much of the NPs' work traversed into the realm of social concerns, I had to account for the fate of a profession that had already staked its own claims in that arena.

In this chapter, I treat the contraction of social work as intrinsic to understanding the story of nursing's expansion. The Grove's mandate of coordination and comprehensive management seemed like the perfect setting to showcase social work's expertise. Moreover, the Grove was mandated to hire social workers—a rarity in outpatient health care. Despite its having all the right organizational conditions, the doors of legitimacy never seemed to open for social work. Exploring how this occurred provides an opportunity to consider the relationship between nursing's professional gains and social work's losses. I do not claim that one is responsible for the other. Rather, I intend to show how the logics and structural conditions that legitimate nursing's expansion are related to those that justified social work's contraction. Physician absence is undoubtedly a necessary condition for nursing's expansion; however, it is not a sufficient one. We must also understand how the NPs' incorporation of social and organizational problems into the clinic came to make more sense than having them resolved within social work.

The Devalued Status of Social Work

Before I had permission to enter the Grove as a researcher, I entered as a volunteer. As a volunteer, I spent ten months understanding the center from the members' perspective. Although I rarely entered the physical clinic during that time,[1] I observed that clinic work was firmly at the core of member life. I knew the names and reputations of the NPs and RNs months before I had the chance to spend any time with them. By contrast, the social workers remained an unknown quantity. Spending my days on the first and second floors with members, I rarely encountered anyone I could even identify as a social worker. I was seldom asked to escort a member to see a social worker; among members, there was no day-to-day gossip about the comings and goings of anyone from that department. Still, while I noted this absence, it was not an observation I found to be especially meaningful. I did not enter the Grove interested in social work. The NPs were my empirical objects of interest. But on my first official day as a researcher, I learned—in the most unambiguous way possible—that the story of the Grove as a nursing organization was also the story of it *not* being a social welfare organization.

I had attended morning meeting in order to give a short but formal introduction to my research. After the meeting, a woman I did not know walked over and introduced herself as one of the Grove's social workers. She was interested in my research and wanted to share an observation of her own. She began to tell me that her work at the Grove "was difficult." She leaned in, with a focused intensity, to say that there were problems "with communication" and "with leadership styles" within the teams. Standing in the hallway, in the midst of her colleagues, she would only speak in vague terms. Months later, during a formal interview, I tried to get her to speak more concretely about her concerns, but she remained guarded, hinting at dissatisfaction but unwilling to say much more. I never did come to know with certainty what was bothering this social worker, but the intensity of her dissatisfaction was something that her colleagues seemed to share. They, however, were willing to voice their diagnosis of the problem, repeatedly, and with a shared articulation: they were social workers, and they struggled for respect in an organization dedicated to health care.

"Social work gets no respect" was SW Rebecca's assessment. While her work with members was challenging, her complaint was not directed toward her clients. Rather, it was an expression of a pervasive feeling that the social workers undeservedly occupied the bottom rung in the Grove's organizational hierarchy. No one, Rebecca felt, treated her expertise as authoritative. She struggled to have her recommendations heard by her team's NP. The OT seemed to veer uncomfortably into her territory. Even the center receptionists wanted to "tell me how to do my job." While it is possible that Rebecca's problems were partly an interpersonal matter, I found her subjective assessment of devaluation to be supported by more than a few objective measures.

In the workplace, the most material measure of value is how much one is paid. When the Grove's social workers compared their salaries to those of people they considered their professional peers, they saw clear evidence that their work was accorded a lower value. SW Rosalie had been working as a master's-trained social worker for more than three decades. Given all the places she had worked, she had a rather blunt assessment of what the Grove paid its social workers. "We're underpaid here; the social workers are definitely underpaid here. . . . I think that's a very important element to introduce to your research." I cannot assess whether these social workers were underpaid relative to social workers in similar organizations. But it is clear that social workers as a group make less than their educations might predict. While the educational credentials required for social worker positions vary by state, all have at least a bachelor's degree, and 45 percent have a master's degree or higher (Salsberg et al. 2017). In 2017, the returns on these investments netted a median yearly income of $47,870 (Bureau of Labor Statistics 2018b). By comparison, in the same year, registered nurses, whose credential for entry could be either an associate's degree or a bachelor's degree, had a median yearly income of $70,000 (Bureau of Labor Statistics 2018a).

While social workers are aware that theirs is not a highly paid profession, such significant differences in pay can start to feel like inequality when contained in the same workplace. One social worker had been pushing the Grove's administration to review her department's salaries. The Grove required its social workers to have a master's degree. She had a suspicion that this credential was not appropriately valued. "I have no way to prove it," she said, "but I think that another department meeting [fewer] educational requirements is probably making more than the social workers." Her campaign had yet to be successful. In the most recent year of her advocacy, the Grove had chosen to raise the wages of the nursing staff rather than those of the social workers.

Money, of course, is not everything. Social workers are not alone in receiving low pay for challenging work. They are joined by kindergarten teachers, day care workers, and home care aides. However, these workers are often the recipients of praise and verbal attestations of their value. While such adulation does not make up for low wages, it is not entirely hollow for those who do the work. For many, such accolades support their own sense of value and moral worth (Diamond 1992; Stacey 2005). From the perspective of the Grove's social workers, their department was rarely on the receiving end of such compensatory praise. SW Deanne offered an illustrative example. "A few years back, our then supervisor nominated every social worker for the excellence award. And we didn't get it. None of us got it. The aides got it. The aides are always being acknowledged and praised. As are the nurses."

The relative devaluation of social work was also visible in the ranks of administration. SW Yvonne was the head of the social work department. When I first interviewed her, I asked her to tell me her official job title. She answered, "Social work supervisor." She then paused before amending with a lowered voice, "There is some inconsistency across the agency with that." The inconsistency she was referring to was that the medical director and the director of nursing were classified as directors. She was a supervisor. This difference was more than semantic. In the Grove's organizational hierarchy, supervisors not only were paid less but also occupied a lower rank than directors. Directors answered to no one but the chief executive officer. Yvonne had a boss. This distinction had not gone unnoticed by the social workers Yvonne supervised. When Yvonne was first hired, Rosalie was openly troubled by what she saw as an explicit devaluation of social work. She specifically pointed out the structurally lower position that Yvonne occupied, observing, "social work is a critical, crucial part that makes this program work cohesively and all the rest of it. But at the top level, we're not recognized."

That social work received "no respect" relative to other departments was a material reality embedded throughout the organization. However, the prevailing belief was that the social workers had no one but themselves to blame. I was not the only one who was perplexed by what the social workers seemed *not* to be doing. A range of staff—from aides to administrators—expressed open dissatisfaction with the social workers' job performance. One NP noted, "I think, theoretically, the role of social worker is [intentional pause] moderately important. . . . But it's colored by the fact that I don't think we've got a particularly strong group of social workers." In explaining the provenance of their dissatisfaction, most staff relied on individual-level theories. There was a pervasive belief that these social workers in particular deserved their lesser status because they had abandoned their traditional realms of work.

A Dereliction of Duty

One of those traditional realms was mental and behavioral health. Social welfare may be the primary terrain for social work; however, mental health has become a close second. Some social workers pursue licensing that allows them to provide clinical counseling services. But even social workers who do not choose a clinical path learn a therapeutic perspective that provides them with expertise in crisis management and client support. Inside the Grove, the link between social work and mental health was not always organizationally visible. At a practical level, the Grove's social worker positions did not explicitly require them to perform clinical work. When I began my fieldwork, none of the team-based social workers was licensed to practice in this way. Instead, the Grove employed a diversely credentialed group of clinicians to provide counseling services. This division of labor was not, in itself, a problem for these social workers. Because of different training and licensure requirements, social workers tend to choose a clinical or nonclinical path early in their careers. Rather, the problem was a symbolic one: the Grove did not recognize social work's expertise in mental health.

As the Grove's census grew, so did the demand for mental health services. To meet that demand, the Grove began employing in-house therapists to provide counseling services. Most recently, they had hired a part-time marriage and family counselor. Rosalie recalled, "We were surprised when we heard that she was being hired." The social workers were not included in that hiring process. They had not been consulted or even informed. Rosalie believed that "behavioral health and social work are under the same umbrella." This connection should have, in her view, given the social workers standing in hiring a mental health provider. On the contrary, social work was unrecognized as having legitimate expertise in mental health.

For some social workers, this lack of recognition was yet another sign of organizational disrespect, but for others, it was a result of the social workers' abdication of professional responsibility. When Yvonne first arrived at the Grove and looked out at the department she inherited, she observed critically, "*Nobody* here is doing clinical work." In her view, instead of attending to the mental and behavioral needs of their members, the social workers were "passing that responsibility off" to other providers. While acknowledging the challenge of large caseloads, she primarily attributed this problem to individual failings. She believed that her departmental charges were simply "uncomfortable with that part of the social work role." She was not alone in that critique.

The primary role of NPs at the Grove was to provide primary care. However, there was another set of NPs who worked across teams to address members' mental health needs. NP Bridgette described her role as consulting with teams on observed behavior changes, with a special focus on members with dementia and Alzheimer's disease. "In older adults," Bridgette explained, "there are so many things that could be causing the psychiatric syndromes; there are so many clinical mimics." Bridgette's professed expertise was more on the medical than the psychological end. "I'm not a psych-mental health nurse. My expertise is in delirium . . . and I have training with dementia." She described her job as providing a "comprehensive look at the patient" that bridged the physical and the psychological. However, she sometimes found the social workers unwilling to be collaborative partners in her bridging role.

Bridgette described a case in which a social worker "really didn't want to have to sit with this patient who was decompensating. But she was the one that was there and had to do it because I wasn't available. She was not happy with me that I couldn't come right that instant to do that. But I'm like, 'I'm sorry. You're a social worker. You can do crisis intervention!' [she laughs] And she did a fine job! She did a great job." Bridgette did not question the social worker's ability—indeed, she praised her as doing "a great job." She did question the social worker's willingness to do the work. For Bridgette, this was the story not just of one social worker but of the department. She noted, "they don't want to do the gero-psych oftentimes because they're so overwhelmed with just getting all their work done." For Bridgette, what the social workers considered "their work" was not in their traditional terrain of mental health.

The social workers seemed to have abdicated their role in mental health on more public stages as well as in individual encounters. In addition to hiring licensed therapists to provide individual therapy, the Grove employed a chaplain and an art therapist. Both of these providers publicly performed their commitment to and expertise in mental health in ways the social workers did not. The chaplain was a resource shared across teams. He did not have the time to regularly attend team meetings, but his presence on team email signaled his commitment to counseling. It was not uncommon for the chaplain to weigh in on member concerns. For example, a team email about a member's use of a motorized wheelchair for long-distance travel elicited a response from the chaplain about how he would "reinforce" the team's concerns by "counseling" the member on safer ways to deal with his feelings of loneliness and isolation. In response to this commitment, the organization recognized his expertise through explicit referrals of members who were struggling with grief, depression, loneliness, or family-level communication.

The chaplain had an acknowledged role in not only directly assisting members but also supporting the organization's role in managing its members.

In addition to the chaplain, the Grove employed an art therapist. As a singular provider, she, like the chaplain, did not attend team meetings but performed her set of commitments over email. She would narratively emphasize progress and include pictures of artwork and poems that had come out of her work with members. Her words did more than summarize a clinical course or outcome; they displayed expertise. As a measure of that expertise, her emails generated responses of encouragement and appreciation for her work with difficult cases. On the organizational stage of email, the art therapist demonstrated her commitment to mental health and was publicly praised for it.

The social workers, by contrast, were not seen as performing this kind of commitment. It may not have been their job to provide formal clinical counseling, but they took few opportunities to publicly perform any expertise in that regard. They did not volunteer to intervene in difficult cases, either over email or in team meetings. Other members of the team referred their own complex problems with members to a therapist, the chaplain, the art therapist, or to an NP. When Yvonne described the social workers as "passing off" clinical work to other providers, she was describing not a division of labor but an abdication of expertise.

This passing off of mental health work occurred in tandem with a passing over of social workers as experts in this area. Bridgette was candid about her own tendency to forget social work's expertise. "I think social work is probably one of those underrecognized professions here. . . . I was guilty of underrecognizing them too. I put together a poster on the interdisciplinary team for mental health and didn't include social work by accident. . . . Somebody asked me at morning meeting, 'Well, where's social work?' I'm like, 'Oh, crap!' [laughs] How can I not put social work in there?" Bridgette's omission was undoubtedly an error rather than an intentional slight. However, this passing over of social work's expertise was reflected in broader organizational beliefs. Without a visible performance of social worker expertise, it became easy to "underrecognize" or forget.

The second of social work's traditional realms of expertise is social welfare. Social work customarily draws much of its expertise about a client's social need through an understanding of social support networks, family dynamics, and community context. Traditionally, social workers develop that understanding through time spent in the field—often through home visits. The Grove's social workers, however, no longer saw this as a routine part of their job. An administrator observed that one social worker in particular wanted "to spend her whole social work career on the phone. You ask her if she's gone out to meet somebody and she says, 'Oh, no, I just talked to them on the phone.' Really?" One of the physicians observed, "The social workers don't want to go out to people's houses.

Plain and simple. They just don't want to go out. Now I'm not a social worker. I don't know anything about being a social worker. But if part of what you do is to try to help manage people's psychosocial issues, wouldn't you want to get a better handle, or as best an idea of what their social setup is?"

Other critiques came in the form of comparisons with other providers. When I asked one NP to describe the role that her social worker played on the team, she responded, "Greta is my social worker," and laughed. The joke was that Greta was not a social worker but the team's OT. For this NP, humor was a way to convey a more sober assessment of the shortcomings of her social worker. She believed the OT knew things about members "because she went out." By contrast, "Social work didn't go out." Another NP was much more effusive. "The OTs are absolutely amazing. I don't know what we'd do without [our OT]. I mean, every-body on the team's important, but the OT is just amazing. . . . She is like my other right arm other than [my primary care nurse] because if there's any issue out in the home, I email the OT or I call the OT and she goes out and assesses it and lets me know what's going on and what needs to be done." When there was a problem in the home, this NP did not call social work. She relied on somebody else.

Organizational valuations of social work ranged from more to less sympa-thetic, but there was a pervasive belief that these social workers, as individuals, had abdicated their responsibility for traditional realms of social work. I can-not rule out individual orientations as an explanation; however, individual-level explanations are incomplete in accounting for group-level trends. It is difficult to imagine that a small group of social workers, whose work was organized by team rather than department, would independently form the same set of profes-sional shortcomings. Organizations get the employees they create, as much as the ones they hire. In my observations, the Grove's social workers were indeed reluctant to do some forms of work. A core part of that reluctance, however, was not from preference but from pressure. Although many saw the social workers as having given up their professional responsibilities, I observed that the Grove pro-vided little opportunity for the social workers to retain them. The social workers' inability to perform ownership of their traditional areas of expertise was less a function of abdication than of structural disinvestment. The withholding of raises and the denial of praise were reflective of an absence of organizational recognition of social work's importance.

Disinvesting in Social Work

Since the Grove first opened its door, it had dramatically increased not only in size but also in complexity. This organizational complexity was matched by that of members. When I spoke with staff who had been there the longest, they often mentioned the higher levels of social and medical acuity of newer members. Everyone in the organization had a story to tell of being asked to do more with less. But the social workers felt they were asked to make do with even less than most. One of their chief problems was large caseloads. When I began my fieldwork, each social worker was responsible for the care of over one hundred members. This was also true of each NP. However, the NPs had the support of a primary care nurse as well as a part-time NP in their day-to-day work. While there were conversations in some quarters about increasing the effectiveness of these supportive players, there was no questioning of the NPs' need for assistance. The medical acuity of the Grove's members legitimated continued investments in the clinic.

The Grove's members, however, also had high levels of social acuity. There were constant emergencies having to do with the basics of food, housing, and safety, all exacerbated by the unchangeable reality that family and community resources were already stretched thin. Everyone at the Grove understood and acknowledged these challenges. However, at the same time that everyone believed that social acuity levels were increasing, investments in social work had decreased. Prior to Yvonne's hiring, the social work supervisor position had been allowed to remain vacant for several years. This vacancy was not an issue with hiring; it was an organizational decision. The position itself had literally been erased from the Grove's organizational chart.[2] This vacancy left the frontline social workers with no one to advocate for their department at the administrative level. Indeed, after she was hired, one of Yvonne's first actions as advocate was getting approval to hire more social workers. Yvonne had her own set of critiques about the department, but she knew that little would change without more people to do the work.

In the face of social acuity, and in the absence of a social work advocate, the default organizational response had been to invest in the expansion of the clinic and to silently disinvest in social work. The social workers were keenly aware of how these constraints affected their work. SW Margaret had been a social worker for almost fifteen years, working primarily in social welfare agencies. She summarized the impact of large caseloads in saying, "With over one hundred members, it's hard to get intimately involved with so many. You lose a lot." What Margaret expressed succinctly, another described in more elaborate form. Natalie was a master's of social work (MSW) student who was completing the second of two social work internships at the Grove. She was only four months into her yearlong placement, but she felt she had been there long enough to know what troubled her about the Grove. For Natalie, high caseloads were more than a challenge; they made "real social work" impossible. "The amount of interactions that I would normally get with a client? I don't necessarily get." Because the social workers did not have enough time, from her perspective, the only thing they could do was make sure "the member is surviving and has basic needs." At the Grove, social work was "all surface work."

In the face of disinvestment, the social workers faced a conundrum: how to reconcile their professional ideals with organizational realities. Although others might have diagnosed the social workers with having given up, the social workers still professed an enduring sense of mission. Margaret opined, "The profession of social work is about empowering people." She spoke passionately about how she tried to do this at the Grove. "Social work is vital. We're the lynchpin for everything. . . . When families call with concerns about medical issues, it is social work that will help members advocate for themselves." Client empowerment is a core feature of social work's professional ethos. Deanne described this feature as the reason she went into social work. "It may sound corny," she said, "but I always felt that I would want my time here on earth to make things better for the rest of the world. I want to be an up-lifter. And I think that you can certainly make that happen through doing [social] work." These were not the words of burned-out cynics. The professional ideals at the heart of social work practice were very much alive in their minds. Yet there was a tension between their professed ideals and the work they did at the Grove. In contrast to their organizational critics, I did not find that the social workers were hiding from work. They were, in fact, quite busy. They spent the majority of their days attending to work that their colleagues may not have valued but that the Grove's structural logics implicitly incentivized: paperwork.

From Social Work to Paperwork

As part of my fieldwork, I attended a range of organizational meetings, including the bimonthly meeting of the social work department. At one such meeting, Yvonne engaged the department in a conversation about what to do for social work month. She asked the social workers to think of ideas "that would pick up our visibility. Something that pushes our work out to the staff." She was, I surmised, in the early stages of a public relations campaign to rescue social work's organizational image. One social worker wondered aloud, "How can we let the staff know what we spend our time doing?" Over the next few minutes of discussion, one suggestion in particular captured their collective imagination: "Why don't we count up how many 1372 forms we do in a month? And display it? Like on a bulletin board?"

Form 1372 had to be completed anytime there was a change in a member's program status. When a member joined or withdrew from the program, changed residence, moved in or out of a nursing home for respite or rehabilitation, transitioned into hospice or long-term nursing care, or died, this form had to be filled out by a social worker. Completing the form accurately generated a cascading set of tasks. If a member moved, the social worker had to verify and document the old and new addresses. When a member went to a nursing home, the social worker had to make phone calls to find an open bed and collect and fax over the appropriate medical documentation. For the Grove's population of members—who were chronically and often acutely ill—1372-defined transitions were a common occurrence. For these social workers, the filling out of form 1372 had become a meaningful visual metaphor for their work.

The filling out of forms was certainly not unique to social work. Health care is a highly bureaucratized endeavor; all manner of providers spend hours documenting clinical encounters, signing prescriptions, and writing referrals. At the Grove, state regulations determined when a medical provider had to see a member, and it set the terms for such encounters by defining what had to be documented. However, in the clinic, the primary content of the work was determined by the provider. Medical encounter forms required a diagnostic category to legitimate payment, but how a diagnosis was appropriately achieved was determined by the clinician. Moreover, state-mandated visits represented only a fraction of clinic work. Paperwork requirements shaped clinic work but did not define it. For the social workers, however, paperwork had come dangerously close to defining the majority of their work.

Others in the organization may have believed the social workers should do more, but they also assessed that filling out paperwork was the primary feature of social work at the Grove. "Their work," according to NP Francesca, "is reviewing the care plan . . . arranging for family meetings, arranging long-term care stays, helping the family and the member with their fiscal management related to eligibility for Medicare and Medicaid. I think that's it." In Bridgette's example of a decompensating member, her evaluation was that the social workers did not perform clinical mental health services because they were busy getting their work done. From her perspective, the social workers had redefined their work as separate from things like clinical work. The social workers' role had been narrowed down to a discrete set of tasks; these tasks were generated almost exclusively by the demands of paperwork.

What accounted for this occupational narrowing was, in part, explained by the paperwork itself. Paperwork is not just a reflection of work; it actively makes some kinds of work visible and others invisible. The Grove was required by the Centers for Medicare and Medicaid Services to use an interdisciplinary team model that included master's-trained, licensed social workers. Despite this requirement, the Grove was still primarily organized around the primacy of medical services. At a fundamental level, the logic of billing made clinic work more highly valued than differently located work. Although the Grove was funded under capitation rather than a fee-for-service model, the physicians and NPs still submitted encounter and diagnostic data that set the level of payment that the Grove would receive for each member. But this data only accounted for medical services.

Much of the actual labor that social workers could have performed was unaccounted for through billing logics and was therefore difficult to both see and protect. The Grove could choose, for example, to go without a social work supervisor for almost three years. Deciding to go without a director of nursing in a nursing organization would have been difficult to imagine; going without a medical director would have been a violation of the Grove's license to operate.[3] The lack of accountability for the broader mission of social work meant that its work could be effectively narrowed down to only those things mandated by the state and captured by form 1372. Little of what social work would name as its expertise was accounted for on this form. What the form captured instead was the state's core concern: making sure the money was being appropriately spent and that it was going to the right place.

While some kinds of paperwork put social work in service to the state, other forms put it in service to other professions. In the mandated six-month member assessments, the social workers had a dual role. They asked some questions related to their professional expertise, such as, "Do you ever have feelings of sadness or depression? Do you sometimes have feelings of anger?" However, social workers were primarily charged with translating the medical plan of care for the members, to make sure they understood and agreed with its contents. The social workers had to obtain and document a member's assent before the care plan could be reviewed by the team and marked as completed by the state's deadline.

Medically driven paperwork mediated the relationship between social worker and member, and thus fundamentally shaped the encounters between them. Going over the care plan was a comprehensive process; it included questions about durable equipment ("It says that you were provided a cane. Does that still work for you?") as well as personal safety ("Do you feel safe in your home environment?"). However, the longest portion of the care plan was the list of diagnoses and prescribed medications. The form of the questions was not about diseases, but about systems. I listened as one of the more rule-based social workers laboriously asked question after question as she peered at the care plan on her computer screen. "Do you have any complaints with your skeletal system? Do you have any complaints with your digestive system? Do you have any complaints with your visual system?" Natalie, the social work intern, described her frustration in being required to go through "pages of medications" that neither she nor the members understood. These organizationally mandated meetings might have served as a time for social workers and members to discuss a fuller range of member concerns. Instead, the social workers were put in charge of asking a set of questions generated out of a medical view of member problems.

In some cases, paperwork explicitly threatened social work's relationship with members. One of the roles that social work filled was to sign and send out denial letters. The Grove was not only the administrative manager of its members' health care needs; it was also their financial manager. Each team had to approve all member services as well as the distribution of durable medical equipment. Often this was a straightforward process based on the evaluation of medical need. However, other requests required the team to balance cost, safety, or a more qualitative assessment of appropriateness. How many pairs of glasses could a member lose before the Grove would stop providing a replacement pair? Should a family's request for more home care hours be approved? These murkier issues were ultimately a team decision. But if a request was denied, a letter of notification was sent out under the social worker's name, not that of the team. If the member had questions about the denial, the person the letter instructed them to contact was the social worker. In this case, it was not a form but a form letter that shaped a potential member encounter. As one social worker put it, "We get left with the dirty work."

Paperwork not only documents work; it produces work. The forms that the social workers were held responsible for did not document traditional social work activities; they generated new forms of social work instead. The social workers spent their days attending to paperwork on behalf of the state and medically oriented providers. Consequently, they had little time left to attend to their profession's traditional realms of expertise. The Grove's disinvestment in social work reflected a broader disinvestment in social problems by state payers.

In having their work so narrowly defined, the social workers were often seen as failing to be good professionals. But the social workers understood their behavior as a realignment of responsibility in the face of competing demands. The Grove's social workers were well aware that they could have done more for members if their time hadn't been so consumed with bureaucratic responsibilities. Most had years—often decades—of experience doing what Natalie would have called "real social work" in other organizations. At the Grove, there seemed to be a host of structural barriers to living out their own ideals of professional practice. Instead of acceding to the impossibility of being good social workers, the Grove's social workers had developed work practices that redefined the scope of their professional responsibilities.

What some saw as refusals to do social work, the social workers experienced as impossibilities. One social worker confided, "Some of us *are* interested in counseling, but with our caseload, there's no way." Several of the social workers surmised that they would not be allowed an opportunity to perform this kind of expertise. Rosalie was one of the social workers with an explicit desire to do counseling work. She had recently invested her own time and money to complete a journaling course with the hopes that she would be able to organize therapeutic support groups at the Grove. In our conversation, however, she tempered her own dreams. In the past, she had not received much administrative support for expanding into more therapeutic realms. She astutely observed, "The Grove needs us to do the bureaucratic work." From Rosalie's perspective, she was not abdicating clinical work; she was barred from investing in it.

That the social workers did not make home visits was, for many, just another example of their personal shortcomings. But Natalie, the social work intern, described it as an organizational rule of thumb: "We're not able to do home visits." In my observation of the entire social work department, I noted that the social workers occasionally went on home visits. But the rule that Natalie had divined was a fairly accurate rendering of the social workers' day-to-day approach: they had turned what could have been a field-oriented profession into an office-based one. They simply did not have the time to go out to the home. For Natalie, this was a sign of the larger failure of the Grove's social workers to meet their profession's standards. When she explicitly compared her work at the Grove to her previous experiences in the field, she observed that it was usually the social workers' knowledge of the home and family milieu that gave them their professional standing. Without that knowledge, the social workers had little that was unique to add to the client's clinical profile.

> At most places of social work, you get this linear kind for thing. [Me: What do you mean by linear?] It's the social worker that follows a client home. You know what's going on in the home. You know what's going on at the medical office. You know what's going on in their personal life. You know what's going on in the psychological piece. You get the whole bio, psych and social compiled together. . . . Versus at the Grove? You get this very small piece in the social work department, *which is unusual for social work*. You get how [members] are in the center. And that's all you get. I guess what I hoped for is that I would get the center plus their home life. Plus their relationship with their family members. Plus a better understanding of what their ailments are and the medical lens. Instead, I get the family system through the lens of someone else's perspective.

For Natalie, "someone else" varied from an intake coordinator in the marketing department to the medication nurse. But often, she observed, it was the NP who "has the bio, psycho, social information. She has the whole gamut. . . . For the most part, the nurses have the biggest grasp on the situation." Natalie had formed a negative evaluation of other social workers' refusal to take on a more traditional social work role. But her own experiences at the Grove quickly matched their behavior. She confided, "I felt I was failing when I first got here. I was fighting to do something more—to have a more challenging experience. But the fight was pushing me even further into what I call the black hole. So I just left it alone. I do what I'm asked now. And I stopped trying to push the issue. I just need to graduate." In the face of organizational disinvestment, even an idealistic intern had learned to accept a diminished role.

At the Grove, social work struggled to remain true to its own professional ideals. Individual social workers professed their commitment to client advocacy, coordination, and problem-solving in the social realm. But most of their work was generated by administrative paperwork rather than direct client appeals. As a result, the purview of the social workers had been reduced to the point where meeting paperwork requirements had become dangerously close to defining the totality of their responsibilities.

The paperwork that structured their days failed to account for traditional social work concerns at the same time that it generated new forms of work that held them accountable to other interests. A significant amount of social work labor was marshaled in support of state concerns as well as the concerns of those who worked inside the clinic. Organizational disinvestment in social work became its own legitimating narrative; social workers were seen not as unable to attend to the social needs of members but as unwilling to do so. Without the resources to support their own ideals about professional social work, the social workers themselves had become participants in narrowing their scope of work.

The NPs' professional openness inside the clinic is only part of the equation of the construction of clinic work; disinvestment in problem-solving outside the clinic is another. The NPs were better able to leverage their knowledge of the social needs of members, in part because the organization had created a situation in which they had more opportunity to garner this expertise as well as more resources to address the needs that they identified. The contraction of social work was not just a matter of dollars and cents; it was embedded in the organizing logic of a health care organization. The Grove's organizational logics remained explicitly medical, despite its mission of comprehensive care. This logic made nursing's location of expertise more compelling than that of social work.

Attention to the everyday constraints of this group of social workers provides a way of understanding the structural and interactional processes through which the clinic, rather than social work, came to make sense as a fitting location for

THE CONTRACTION OF SOCIAL WORK

social and organizational problems. A better understanding of organizational sense-making provides not only a static description of the current division of labor but also a dynamic portrait of the institutional practices through which these divisions are reproduced. Because occupational legitimacy is recursively embedded in everyday action, it serves as both an effect and a cause.

The Grove is just one organization, but there are links between what happened inside its walls and broader negotiations beyond them. There are many explanations for social work's struggles to protect both its work and its status as an occupation. Social work, like nursing, is a predominately female occupation. Scholars have noted that evaluations of skill, status, and occupational value are gendered (England 2010; England and Folbre 1999; Padavic and Reskin 2002; Ridgeway 1997; Sandelowski 2000; Stanek Kilbourne et al. 1994). Social work's gendering as female may delegitimize its claims for expertise and value.

Other scholars might point to social work's struggle to operationalize successful professionalization strategies. The profession has, for example, been able neither to establish occupational closure (Freidson 1988c) nor to convince others that it possesses its own body of abstract knowledge (Abbott 1988). These explanations are undoubtedly part of the larger puzzle. But there is something other than the strategies of professional advocates that requires attention. At the same time that social work's fortunes have fallen, nursing's have risen—maybe not to the heights to which it aspires, but undoubtedly further than current theories would lead one to expect.

At the Grove, the fate of the social workers seemed less about choices in an arena of competition and more the result of the delegitimization of social problems. The social workers were fighting a battle they seemed destined to lose. Social workers repeatedly explained their embattled position by pointing out the fact that the Grove "was a nursing organization" rather than a social service organization. There was a sense not only that they did not have time to do the kind of social work they were trained to do but also that there was less room to conceive of solutions that came from outside the clinic.

It was Margaret who observed, "Social workers used to do discharge planning; but [nurses] have taken that over too." In the 1980s, it was originally social work that elevated discharge planning and medical case management to a professional activity. Today, medical social workers have found themselves vying for this work with both differently credentialed RNs and a diverse range of uncredentialed case workers. Margaret's observation of losing discharge planning to nursing was a general one, but she could just as easily have been talking about the Grove. The Grove employed an RN, not a social worker, to manage member transitions home from hospitals and rehabilitation facilities. The supportive work of making these transitions work smoothly was done by yet another group of nurses. It was primarily the NPs on each team who counseled families about changes in members' mental or physical status and reassessed for increased support.

Since the late 1960s, the state has remained willing to invest in health care even as it has been increasingly unwilling to invest in social welfare. In pragmatic terms, the state has become the primary payer for medical problems at the same time that it has withdrawn as the primary payer for social problems. At the Grove, the state's disinvestment in social problems was manifested in organizational disinvestment in social work. In the face of that disinvestment, the social workers often felt compelled to disinvest in their traditional arenas of work, which only served to legitimate their low valuation.

Nursing has a history of opening new professional doors by arguing for its utility. Nursing advocates identified state and organizational needs and argued that nurses were both willing and able to be a professional solution. However, the fate of social work might be seen as a cautionary tale of such an approach. At the Grove, social work became almost entirely defined by its utility to the organization in meeting the demands of the state. The social workers had become women of the organization in ways that threatened to preclude their championing the needs of their clients.

THE MISRECOGNITION OF
SOCIAL PROBLEMS

A clearer view of the challenges faced by the Grove's social workers provides a better understanding of the hurdles faced by the profession at large. State disinvestment in social problems grounds the devaluation of social work as a profession. This clarity, however, may be of little interest to anyone who is not a social worker. There are always winners and losers in professional contests. If the Grove's members were getting their needs met by others—whether it be NPs, chaplains, or OTs—it's not readily apparent how this devaluation might impact anything other than the professional aspirations of social workers.

In this chapter, I argue that there are consequences for relocating problems from one terrain to another. The tools found in the clinic may not be the same as those located outside it. Moreover, not all social work concerns are necessarily taken up by those best positioned as advocates. At the Grove, social concerns were addressed both by those with recognized credentials and by those without them. "Anyone," it seemed, could do social work. When anyone is perceived as able to do social work, clients may lose an ally with the organizational power to advocate on their behalf. In this chapter, I illustrate that the relocation of social problems is more than a cosmetic rearrangement of who does what; it has implications for our understanding of what constitutes those problems and what we envision as the available arsenal of solutions.

Geographies of Urgency

The contraction of social work was legitimated through state investment in medical problems and disinvestment in social problems. These material realities shaped not just the content of work but how it unfolded across time and space. The primacy given to medical concerns created geographies of urgency within the clinic. Problems brought there were often solved quickly—according to clinic time. The need to triage urgent complaints meant that the doors of the clinic were always open. Social work often found itself out of step with this sense of urgency. In addition to material disinvestments in the social work department, the phenomenon of being "out of step" created a legitimating situation such that the rejection of social work solutions came to seem reasonable to both members and staff.

The Grove occupied three floors of its four-story building. The third floor was mostly office space; members largely spent their days on the first and second floors. Although each floor had a large multipurpose room for member activities, the second floor was the heart of center life. The second floor held a game room, three rooms for arts and crafts, and a chapel, as well as the office of the chaplain and the physical therapy gym. It also housed the clinic. The close proximity of activities to the clinic was not insignificant. For a population with mobility challenges, it mattered that the clinic was accessible without much in the way of physical barriers. Many members could get there on their own. For members who needed staff or volunteer assistance to make the trip, the accessibility of the clinic was less a function of location than it was of organizational priority. In a medically fragile population, the request to go to the clinic was taken seriously.

This contrasted rather sharply with the geography of social work. Instead of being located in the heart of center life, social workers were stationed in offices on the third floor. The ease of getting to the clinic was proportional to the difficulty of getting to the third floor. All members required an escort on the elevators, regardless of physical ability. At organizationally defined moments, such as when members went to lunch, aides would efficiently shuttle large numbers of members from one floor to another. Outside these moments, traveling between floors was much more difficult. Finding an escort willing to wait for an elevator with enough room for a wheelchair or walker was not a simple matter; it was a significant time investment that many staff actively avoided. Because of the demands on staff time, a significant part of my job as a volunteer was to shuttle members to the few recreational activities that took place on the third floor, such as the Thursday afternoon computer class or the Wednesday morning poetry group. Occasionally, however, a member asked for my help in getting to social work.

One afternoon, Ms. Rose waved me over and asked me to take her to see her social worker. She was having a problem with an aide at her assisted living facility and wanted her social worker to do something about it. With a walker, Ms. Rose could move independently. Her chief reason for flagging me down was to operate the elevator. When the elevator had delivered us to the third floor, I accompanied Ms. Rose down the hallway toward her social worker's office. She did not need any help finding the office, but I suspected she might need a return escort sooner than she expected. There is no receptionist or waiting room for social work. The two of us went straight to SW Rebecca's door. The door was closed; Ms. Rose knocked. Rebecca opened the door, but only a crack, so that we could not see in. She did not say anything, but met Ms. Rose's eyes with a look of question.

"Rebecca. I need to talk to you about my aide."

"Ms. Rose, I can't help you right this moment. I'm busy speaking with another member. You are welcome to wait. But I'm not sure I'll have time to speak with you today. You should call and make an appointment."

Waiting was not a novel experience for Ms. Rose. She waited all the time in the clinic. I had watched her wait for an RN or NP for up to an hour on multiple occasions. But waiting for social work was not quite the same experience. In the absence of a waiting room, Ms. Rose sat down to wait on the single chair placed outside Rebecca's door. In that quiet stretch of hallway, there were no compatriots with whom to pass the time. I tried to make polite conversation as I stood beside her, but I was a poor substitute for the hustle and bustle of the clinic. Our waiting also held little hope for resolution. In the clinic, Ms. Rose knew someone would have to hear her out. Rebecca had made no such promises. The minutes tick by fairly slowly under these conditions. I was not surprised when Ms. Rose soon decided she had waited long enough and asked me to take her back to the second floor.

Unplanned trips to social work almost always ended in frustration. The investment of time and effort—which was considerable for members with less mobility—often yielded little. After witnessing this scenario multiple times, I began to take note of how infrequently members spoke of needing to see a social worker. One or two experiences like that of Ms. Rose were enough to learn that one could not just drop in on a social worker. Members saw their social workers every six months, when the state mandated a visit, but social work was not a resource they could easily access for their own purposes.

Social work's inaccessibility was not a literal truth. Members could make appointments. But it was a relative truth—relative to the clinic. The clinic functioned more like an emergency room than an outpatient clinic. The need to triage was institutionally recognized. Even if an NP or primary care nurse could not see you, some kind of licensed provider had to listen to your concern in order to gauge its medical importance. Sitting in the waiting room could itself be a useful way to get a problem solved. Members who sat long enough might find themselves able to shout out their concerns directly when the NPs or primary care nurses came out. Sometimes, they were gratified with a quick waiting-room consultation. At other times, the NP or RN might at least hear the complaint and reassure the member by saying, "I've added you to my list for tomorrow. Come back and we can talk about it." Members may not always have gotten the response they wanted, but they always got a response. The one thing they were never asked to do was to call and make an appointment.

When social workers used the language of appointments, they were employing an ordering of time that made little organizational sense to members. The clinic did not run on appointments. The NPs and primary care nurses created lists of members to see in a given week. The aides were given these lists and brought members to the clinic in no particular order. Those who were being monitored closely may have been instructed to "come every day for the next two weeks" for vitals. But no one was ever told, "You have a clinic appointment at ten a.m." Some saw it as another sign of the Grove's failure to run like a doctor's office, but there were real obstacles to an appointment-based system. The timing of center visits varied depending on alterations in a van driver's route, a member's illness, or a competing specialist appointment. There were also other health-related activities that had to be accommodated, such as time in the physical therapy gym or a group therapy session. Flexibility in the clinic allowed members to have flexibility in how they navigated their days at the center.

The logic of appointments also made little organizational sense to staff. Staff, like members, preferred more immediate forms of communication and problem-solving. For many, this immediacy was achieved by email, but for some workers, the ability to drop in for face-to-face conversation was key. For example, the Grove's aides were the eyes and ears of the organization in terms of changes in members' behavior and functionality. Some of the aides also provided home care to members, positioning them to relay information gathered from both the center and home. But in order for this information to be useful, they had to be able to communicate it effectively. As these were not desk jobs, email was not their preferred way of doing so. As direct care providers, their work was tied to the locations and rhythms of members. Therefore, typically, when an aide wanted to relay a problem about a member, the aide relayed it via face-to-face communication rather than email. Just as was true for members, a door somewhere in the clinic was always open to their concerns. To attempt to speak with a social worker was to encounter some of the same obstacles that the members faced: finding the time to travel up to the third floor only to potentially face a closed door.

The urgency of the clinic was not just about physical accessibility. It was equally about response time. One of the key complaints about the social workers was that they did not respond quickly. One NP explained that it was a problem that "the social worker is up on the third floor. Somebody needs to find a social worker, and it's so much trouble. . . . It's just not accessible to the members. . . . I could call the social worker. And she'll say, 'Have them sit out there' [in the clinic waiting room]. And *maybe* she'll come down. And it's frustrating because maybe if you call and then they're not at their desk then you're left with this thing to do." The social workers did not act quickly enough for some clinic staff. They often did not act quickly enough for members.

It was a relatively quiet afternoon in the clinic. I was sitting in RN Joanne's office when we heard a voice. "Joanne! Joanne!" Joanne looked at me with her uncanny ability to both be expressionless and speak volumes. Ms. Gillespie walked through Joanne's open door and sat down. Joanne opened the conversation.

"How are you, Ms. Gillespie?"

"Not good. Not good. I don't feel well. And my blood pressure is two hundred."

Ms. Gillespie's vitals were just the prelude to what she had really come to talk about: food stamps. "Food stamps" is the term most people use when referring to the federal Supplemental Nutrition Assistance Program (SNAP). This program is one of the few means-tested benefits that adults can qualify for without dependent children. Ms. Gillespie had been a longtime SNAP recipient, but for the first time in twenty years, she had been kicked off its rolls. She was in a panic that had quickly turned into anger.

The clinic was her second stop. Her first stop had been social work. I do not know what transpired between Ms. Gillespie and her social worker, but whatever had occurred, it had not alleviated her worries. She had arrived in Joanne's office with her voice raised in frustration, punctuating her words by waving the letter she had received from the county. "I just got a letter from a case worker—somebody that I've never seen or talked to—saying that I'm being kicked off food stamps!" She handed Joanne the letter; Joanne quickly scanned through its words before responding.

"Hmmm. I cannot say exactly what this means. But it looks like you needed to send in some kind of paperwork to recertify your eligibility."

"But I've never had to do that before!"

"I know. It must be frustrating."

"I tried talking to that social worker," Ms. Gillespie began, "but she doesn't know what she's talking about."

Joanne kept her own voice low and steady as she responded. "I'm not sure what the social worker can help you with, but what I can do is have the kitchen send home some food to tide you over. Some milk. Cereal. Bread. Okay?" "Okay,"

Ms. Gillespie answered, her voice lowering to match Joanne's. After Ms. Gillespie left, Joanne sent an email to the kitchen to request that a box of food be sent home with Ms. Gillespie. The email was the documented, formal request, but Joanne walked downstairs to speak with the kitchen staff directly to make sure it happened by day's end. When she returned to her office, she sent off another email. Since she could see Ms. Gillespie's agitation was making her feel unwell, she wrote to transportation to request that her van driver take Ms. Gillespie home early. The social worker would undoubtedly be the one to deal with Ms. Gillespie's SNAP recertification. But it was Joanne who was both easy to reach and quick to act. The immediate satisfaction Ms. Gillespie had not found in social work she had found in the clinic.

For members as well as staff, the logic of medical necessity created geographies of urgency. As long as they appeared in the clinic, a wide range of problems were triaged and treated as potential emergencies. Moreover, the clinic had comparatively more resources than social work with which to both listen and act. The ability to have your concerns met quickly seemed to have few downsides. There was also a legitimate critique to be made about the difficulty members had in accessing their social workers. However, when problems are relocated to landscapes of medical urgency, there are implications for the universe of possible solutions.

The Impossibility of Social Work Solutions

Just as I had the opportunity to watch a new set of physicians find their place in a nursing organization, I had the chance to watch a new group of social workers do the same. When she became the new social work supervisor, one of SW Yvonne's first departmental interventions was to hire more social workers. Almost seeming to take the clinic as her model, she was experimenting with a system in which a part-time social worker would support the work of the full-time social worker on each team. SW Lisette was hired to fill one of those part-time positions. I watched as Lisette oriented to the Grove and its team-based approach to care. I also observed her adjustment to the limited role of social work on the team. The primary location of this adjustment was within weekly team meetings. Lisette mostly chose to sit silently through these meetings; this was not an unreasonable choice given her status as a new employee. However, there was one meeting early in her tenure in which I watched her not only learn the circumscribed role of social work at the Grove but also come face-to-face with the difficulty of offering social work solutions in a landscape of urgency.

Because it was Friday, NP Norah's team meeting was scheduled to happen right after morning meeting. But Norah was out of the office. In her absence, NP Francesca had stepped in to move the team through their agenda. Prior to the meeting, there had already been a flurry of emails about a complaint from the transportation department. Ms. Reed was never ready when her transport arrived to pick her up. This was more than a hassle; it was an expense. The type of assistance Ms. Reed needed could not be accomplished by the Grove's van drivers. She was listed as a "two-man assist" and could not be accommodated by the solo driver who went out in the van. The Grove had to hire a medical transportation company in order to get Ms. Reed to the center. If she was not ready when they arrived, the company rescheduled the transport—an additional service for which the Grove was billed. The team had been emailed; they had a problem they needed to solve.

The team's conversation about Ms. Reed was freewheeling. SW Margaret, the team's full-time social worker, believed the transportation company might have been coming a few minutes early on some days, which explained why Ms. Reed wasn't ready. The primary care nurse thought the problem might be with the family's struggle to keep to a scheduled routine. A center aide offered her firsthand observation that Ms. Reed "just eats slow." But it was PT Abby who highlighted what eventually came to define the crux of the problem. "I thought," Abby said with a deep frown, "we had moved her from the second floor down to the first floor? If she's on the first floor she can be a Grove transport." Switching Ms. Reed's transportation from a contracted company to the Grove would not necessarily solve the problem of her not being ready, but the team might be able to work more effectively toward a solution if they had direct control. The Grove's drivers were also more inclined to be flexible; they might wait a few extra minutes for a member who fell behind schedule.

The first thing the team needed before they could move forward was better information. They called the transportation coordinator into the meeting, who said, "As far as I know, they are still getting Ms. Reed from the second floor. . . . I need confirmation that she has a first-floor setup before I can switch her to a Grove transport." Abby immediately volunteered to go out to the home. Her willingness was partly motivated by her frustrations with transportation. Abby had helped to orchestrate moving Ms. Reed's sleeping arrangements to the first floor; she was keen to figure out why her recommendations had seemingly been ignored. "If the team said she wasn't safe being brought down from the second floor . . . why is transportation still doing it?"

Abby's desire to make a home visit was echoed in an unexpected corner. As soon as Abby stated her intention, Lisette said, "I'd like to go with you." Abby made eye contact with Lisette but made no comment. After a brief pause, Francesca asked when Abby planned to go out. "This weekend. It needs to be a surprise if we are going to see what's really going on." At that, Lisette had nothing to say. Francesca then proceeded to crystallize the plan. "So PT is going to make a home visit to see what's going on. Then it sounds like it's time for a family meeting. We may need to lay down the law with this family."

As I watched this encounter, it occurred to me that Abby and Francesca were each, in her own way, doing what could have been the work of the social worker. Abby was making a home visit, not to do a PT assessment, but "to see what's going on." Francesca decided that a family meeting needed to happen and set the tone for what that meeting needed to accomplish. But in all this seeming social work activity, the voice of an actual social worker was sidelined. Lisette's request to make a home visit was met with silence by both the PT and the NP. Part of that silencing was achieved by the simple act of declaring that the home visit had to happen *now*.

Once again, social work was out of sync with the urgency that was commonplace at the Grove. Although the problem with transportation had been percolating for months, once it came to the clinical setting of team meeting, it suddenly seemed urgent. The visit needed to be "a surprise" for the family. It also needed to happen in less than twenty-four hours, which, in this case, happened to fall on a Saturday. There was no attempt to accommodate either the rhythms of social work or the practical constraints of a staff member who worked part-time. Lisette also received an important lesson about the role of social work at the Grove: her role was limited to paperwork and carrying out tasks that the team had orchestrated. Although Francesca had determined that a family meeting was the next step, one of the social workers would be tasked with organizing it. I wondered how the conversation about Ms. Reed might have proceeded if it had appeared in a different landscape of expertise, outside the geographies of urgency in which clinic concerns took shape.

Some of the social workers had their own answer to this question. SW Emma was another new hire. At twenty-eight years old, she was new to the profession as well as to the Grove. Perhaps because she had the support of a social work supervisor—and had less than a year on the job—Emma did not share the same experience of devaluation as many in her department. She did, however, share the view of her colleagues that social work not only carried out different tasks but also offered a different disciplinary perspective. "In our team meetings when everyone would bring up their points [about members], I just look at it differently. To me? I see what they're saying, but to me the solution seems different than what a medical model solution would be." She offered an example of how her perspective as a social worker made a difference in the case of Ms. Bunn.

Emma described Ms. Bunn as someone who was "in total care." Ms. Bunn needed direct assistance with bathing, dressing, and eating, as well as medication administration. Although home care aides provided considerable help, the bulk of that care was provided by Ms. Bunn's family. But the family was inconsistent with providing this care. According to Emma, Ms. Bunn's care plan was not being executed. "I mean, some people have to get their insulin. That's something that's valid. Her [adult diapers] were not being changed; she was coming into the center dirty. We actually ended up making a protective service report [to the state]."

These were serious problems that could not be ignored. According to Emma, the medical providers on the team had been holding the threat of the nursing home over the family. However, in Emma's telling of the story, she employed a different approach. She listened to and acknowledged the family's fears of nursing home placement. "The reality is the nursing homes in this area of the city are not the greatest." But she also validated how much they were doing. "I think it's easy to kind of get down on the family for not doing enough for their family members. But instead you can look at it like, 'Wow, you're really doing a lot.' In any other situation, this woman would already be in a nursing home." In hearing them out, she was able to build a different relationship with the family. "It actually ended up working really well. She's been getting her insulin and everything. So kind of coming at it from that way, instead of saying, 'You have to give the insulin, you're not doing these things correctly'—a lot of times it comes across as they're doing a terrible job as caregivers." Emma recognized the seriousness of the situation, but getting to the best solution required its removal from the clinic's geography of urgency and into the one in which the family lived. The ability to see things from their perspective and to not focus solely on the medical intervention was, for Emma, "something that social workers do a lot."

If the legitimacy of the NPs was predicated on their position within the medical encounter, Emma's words illustrate that the potential power of social work lay in specifically remaining outside of it. The logic of medical necessity that legitimated resource use at the Grove could also be used to threaten the agency of members and their families. Emma saw social work's role as advocating for members by giving voice to solutions that could not be found in the clinic. This ideal was not unique to Emma, but was inculcated by her profession. SW Flora described the role of social work as "advocating for those who can't advocate for themselves—sometimes hearing what [clients] are saying even when they're not saying it."

Emma may have felt that there was room for this role at the Grove. Many of the social workers did not. Flora followed up her description of what social workers did with a description of the hurdles she faced in doing so at the Grove. "I spend a lot of time standing my own ground as an advocate for myself and my profession so folks can realize that [my approach] is not wrong, it's just different. That takes quite a bit of time. I spend a lot of time developing respect for my profession." Some social workers located this difficulty within the Grove's organizational DNA. Margaret opined there was sometimes a conflict of interest between the mandate to care for members and that of supporting their autonomy: "I think sometimes we get *too* involved in people's lives." Margaret continued, "The profession of social work is about empowering people. You don't hear a lot about that here." The Grove had an obvious organizational interest in wanting care provision to run smoothly. At the center, this was not much of a problem. However, when it came to locations outside the center, there was sometimes friction between how members and families lived and what was easiest for the Grove to manage.

For some social workers, the Grove's health care focus was part of the problem. They believed that nursing's imperative to care for dependent populations was sometimes at cross-purposes with supporting individual autonomy. The other problem was more insidious. Margaret noted, "We are their health care provider and their insurer; these are competing interests." She was not alone in linking the health care imperative to an overly interventionist orientation to members' lives. Half the Grove's social workers shared Margaret's observation that sometimes the logic of medical necessity created a sense of urgency around problems that in other settings might simply be considered the vicissitudes of everyday life. This point of view, however, struggled to be heard with equal weight in an organization geared toward health care.

A case that illustrates that struggle involved Ms. Bowie. Ms. Bowie was a member who lived in an apartment building staffed with home care aides who provided personal care services to residents. Ms. Bowie lived on a floor with residents categorized as independent. She had assistance with the activities of daily living, but she retained the right to make her own decisions. Although the Grove and the building were organizationally and fiscally separate, they found it mutually beneficial to work with one another. As part of this working relationship, the building's management had a direct line of communication to the Grove. The building had used this direct line to relay a problem with Ms. Bowie: her cooking. According to the building's aides, Ms. Bowie's cooking produced "a strong smell" and a lot of smoke. On more than one occasion, she had set off her apartment's smoke alarm. In a setting where few residents actually cooked—most relied on boxes from the frozen-food aisle or premade meals from the kitchens of friends and family—Ms. Bowie had become a problem for the building. In turn, she had become a problem for the Grove.

As Ms. Bowie's team discussed the problem, the overtly subjective complaints about strong smells receded to the background, while the more objective complaints about the production of smoke became the focal point. "Is she," the NP asked, "safe to cook?" Although Ms. Bowie did not have a diagnosis of Alzheimer's or advanced dementia, a behavioral health clinician raised questions about possible impairments. SW Rebecca countered that there was no evidence that this was the problem with her cooking. "If she is frying something, it might smoke up the place, not because she's causing a fire, but just because that's what frying does." The social worker's reframing of the problem, however, was not able to shift the conversation. The consensus began to form that the problem with Ms. Bowie's cooking was most likely a problem with Ms. Bowie; she just might be unsafe to cook alone. The OT suggested removing the knobs from the stove and leaving them with the building's aides. Ms. Bowie could still cook, but she would have to ask for assistance—and thus accede to supervision—when she did so.

No decision about Ms. Bowie was made that day, but the narrative surrounding the problem had seemingly been set. Ms. Bowie's cooking had become a problem that required a clinical intervention. The social worker was the only one not in agreement with this view. After the meeting, I asked Rebecca about its outcome. Her perspective was that the team often seemed unable to see things from the member's point of view. "Everybody is too quick to blame everything on her . . . having behavioral issues and burning down the place. But any woman in a kitchen—cooking fish, frying chicken—has set off a smoke alarm."

The social worker's move to normalize member problems was in direct contrast to the medicalizing moves of others. Rebecca asked the team to imagine Ms. Bowie as "any woman in a kitchen." However, this view of Ms. Bowie was summarily rejected. I also had questions about the solution on offer. Having spent time in the homes of members who lived in supportive settings, I wondered just how accommodating an aide would be to the need to supervise Ms. Bowie's cooking. The aides had already been unequivocal about their aversion to the smells her cooking produced. Moreover, the way aides organized their work did not include supervising an activity such as cooking. Ms. Bowie cooked as much for pleasure as for sustenance. Doing it herself, according to her own routines or lack thereof, was undoubtedly why she wanted to make some of her own meals. Her desire for creativity might find itself at odds with an aide's need for efficiency. Supervising resident cooking was also not the kind of essential work that a supervisor might privilege; an aide might not always find time for an "extra" activity that they might assess as a lower priority than assisting with bathing, toileting, or warming up a microwaveable dinner for other residents.

In offering this case, my intent is not to criticize the specifics of the team's decision. As someone with no clinical training, I am not equipped to do so. However, it is illustrative of the ways in which social work's perspective was not treated as equivalent to those from inside the clinic. Even when the problem did not concern a diagnosis or an explicitly medical intervention, the social worker's perspective, far from taking precedence, was not even acknowledged. Once the aides' complaints had been transformed into a clinical problem, one realm of solutions was opened while another seemed forever closed. The embattled place of social workers not only had consequences for their status as professionals but also impacted how member problems were understood.

For the social workers, the ability to understand a situation from the member's perspective was a professional ideal as well as a product of professional training. A key part of that perspective was an attention to diversity. Emma believed that her training as a social worker gave her a different set of resources through which to understand the perspective of the Grove's almost entirely African American patient population. "I think we play a really big part in understanding the diversity in our population. You know, the majority of our team is Caucasian and female. It's almost as if we speak a different language; it's missing what a lot of our population is—what they're saying." Emma herself identified as a white woman; however, she believed that as a social worker, she had the professional training to differently see and consider how factors such as race, culture, and poverty impacted the Grove's encounters with its members.

> As a social worker, you're paying attention to, it's not just the medical side, but it's everything else that people bring to the table and how that kind of plays in. I thought I'd just put that in your brain. I think that's one thing that the social workers are kind of in charge of: looking at the cultural issues as well as the economic. There's no question about that. Also, for bringing up that people might be looking at the problem, not from a medical standpoint, but from what it means to their religion or their family or their culture or their race, that sort of thing.

As a demographic fact, the social work department was more diverse than the NPs. All the NPs were white, whereas only half the social work department identified as such. This relative diversity was also noted by other social workers as a distinguishing feature. Rebecca opined, "I don't think the white people here always understand that the members are old. They've lived through the war [of racial discrimination]. They don't always trust white people." She believed these members "came to social work" to speak with social workers like herself who were not white.

It is not entirely clear whether the individual backgrounds of the social workers is what mattered most. The Grove's NPs were exclusively white, but the broader nursing staff, including the primary care nurses, were almost exclusively not—whether they identified as African American, hailed from the Caribbean, or claimed a nationality from the continent of Africa. The two full-time clinic physicians were white, but both the medical director and the longtime part-time physician were African American. However, what Emma described was a difference in a *professional* perspective that was attuned to culture. What she seemed to be articulating was the difficulty of accounting for diversity when the tools one brings to the encounter are medical ones, no matter how broadly one defines them.

Losing a Potential Advocate

The social workers believed that they offered a perspective that was different from the medical world of the clinic. They argued that their ability to see the world from the member's perspective gave them a unique role on the team. The practical difficulty with basing their expertise on understanding the member's perspective was that a great many other people at the Grove did so as well. Members had the ears of van drivers, receptionists, aides, recreation assistants, and administrative assistants. In some ways, these workers, collectively, might have had the best understanding of the member's worldview because they often lived in the same neighborhoods as members. The Grove's rules of eligibility required that members come from a specific set of zip codes. Many of the Grove's administrative and support staff not only were African American as a demographic category but also shared the same zip codes as the members. Some had known members prior to meeting anew at the Grove. Others went to the same churches, knew the same people, and remembered the same local histories.

While many of these workers did occasionally advocate for members, one of the nonclinical departments that came dangerously close to treading on the professional toes of social work was marketing. The social worker who suspected that staff in another department with fewer credentials made more money than the social workers had been referring to the marketing department. The possibly lower salaries of social work compared to marketing had, perhaps, a rather pedestrian explanation. The Grove would not be the only organization where those who brought in the money, so to speak, earned more than those who performed credentialed work. At the Grove, however, this disparity was organizationally visible in the starkest way possible: it was not uncommon for workers to effectively get promoted out of social work and into marketing.

In addition to the master's-trained social workers, the Grove had once chosen to hire case workers without these credentials to help the social workers by doing the legwork for difficult cases.[1] These workers found that no matter how well they did their jobs, there was little room for advancement in social work. However, they were able to raise their salaries as well as their level of workplace autonomy by moving into marketing. Two of the three intake coordinators in marketing had taken their first positions in the social work department as case managers. SW Rosalie observed that the only way they could advance was to leave. "They come to our department and then we lose them."

The marketing department presented another problem for social work. It was not only the workers who migrated to marketing but also the work. Sadna was one of the marketing intake coordinators who had started in social work. As a case worker, her role had been to do the more time-intensive work that the social workers did not have time to do. One of her cases was Mr. Carver. Before becoming a member at the Grove, Mr. Carver had fallen prey to a predatory mortgage loan. He had been near the end of his working life but was not quite ready for retirement. He made the decision to invest in additional job training. Like many working-class men, he had little savings, but he did have an asset: his house. He took out an eight-thousand-dollar mortgage to pay for the training. But before he was able to make much use of it, he had a disabling stroke that left him with weakness on his left side and a seizure disorder. Mr. Carver had taken out the loan as a bet against future work that he would never be able to do. In the interim, the original eight-thousand-dollar loan had ballooned into a forty-thousand-dollar debt. The lender had moved to foreclose on his house.

"I don't usually worry," Mr. Carver confided to me. "But I was up all weekend worrying about my house. I don't have nowhere else to go." This conversation was spurred by his receiving yet another foreclosure notice in the mail. Mr. Carver was in a battle to save his house, and he had few resources of his own to bring to the fight. Someone had to help Mr. Carver find legal counsel. Someone had to try to negotiate with the lender. Someone had to reach out to Mr. Carver's daughter, whose name was still on the deed of the house. This was the kind of time-intensive case that went to the Grove's case workers.

When Sadna moved from social work to marketing, it was not clear who would do this work. Mr. Carver, however, did not pay much attention to job titles. When he got his latest foreclosure notice, he did not just share his worries with me; he continued to share them with Sadna. When he called her, she reassured him, telling him "not to worry about it" because she was taking care of it. When I asked Sadna about continuing to help Mr. Carver, she explained, "I took a few cases like Mr. Carver with me when I left social work." It would have been difficult, she said, to hand such a complicated case to another person. Moreover, "the social workers don't really have time for that kind of work."

Sadna's decision to continue to help Mr. Carver was partly a personal one. But her individual decision mirrored the informal social work role the marketing department played more broadly. This role could be seen most clearly during the enrollment process. The marketing staff were the first point of contact for prospective enrollees. The initial conversation began over the telephone and culminated in a home visit. When I traveled with marketing staff to evaluate member eligibility, I was surprised to witness conversations that looked a lot less like a marketing pitch and more like a clinical assessment. One of the marketing coordinators described the role as "bringing the person back" to the assessment committee that decided on enrollment. In the encounters I witnessed, the marketing staff took this role seriously. They asked about family support, took a medical history, and recorded observations on the condition of the home.

The initial information recorded by marketing was used to flag potential problem areas and to help decide whether a separate visit by occupational therapy or home care was necessary. In many cases, however, they were the *only* members of staff who visited the home before approval. While other providers would eventually assess the person at the center, the marketing staff were positioned to know things that went beyond self-report. They had seen the member navigate in his or her own surroundings, not just in the accessible architecture of a medical center. They could also see how the member interacted with family, as well as observe which family was or was not at home. They may not have had enough information to know the whole case, but they could competently paint the outlines of it. Because the marketing staff had firsthand information, their reports about social context were treated as more reliable than those of the social worker, whose assessments were done at the center. As the first point of contact with members and their families, the marketing department also functioned as a customer service liaison for members after enrollment. It was often they who were asked to translate member concerns across the boundaries of race, economics, and culture. In more ways than one, the marketing department seemed to be performing social work.

In previous chapters, I illustrate how members and staff would stand in the physical and virtual doorways of the NPs. Whether an individual NP was perceived to be good at her job or not, the NPs as a group were treated as the experts for complex member problems. The social workers had the opposite problem. There often seemed to be a lack of recognition that what the social workers possessed qualified as expertise. This ethos allowed "uncredentialed" workers like the marketing staff to use common sense and a caring sensibility to act as social workers. The Grove did recognize the social milieu as an arena of work, but it delegitimated the social workers as possessing any particular expertise within it. The social workers were losing domains of work not only to differently credentialed workers but also to those with no credentials at all.

It may seem less important who addresses such problems, as long as they are addressed. Yet just as it mattered whether member problems were located inside or outside the clinic, it potentially made a difference who members turned to as an advocate in the social terrain. While many workers were recognized as sources of information, not everyone was recognized as an equal in terms of making decisions. Although the social workers sometimes felt disrespected when receptionists and marketing staff felt empowered to tell them "how to do their jobs," these other workers did not have the institutional power to influence the primary decision makers on the clinical team: the medical providers.

Some members did call the marketing department to express their dissatisfaction with the Grove's care. The marketing department took their duty to relay member concerns to the team seriously. However, some in marketing were frustrated by their powerlessness to intervene. Although marketing and social work staff did not always see eye-to-eye, in many ways, they shared a similar set of critiques about the Grove. They too had identified the Grove's level of "intrusiveness" into the personal choices of members as a problem. "It certainly is easier to care for people if you can control what they do," one marketing coordinator observed. "But they have a choice about how they want to live their lives." The marketing staff could relay the concerns of members, but they were not clinicians. They were not a part of the clinical team. Marketing had few formal mechanisms through which to advocate for members and their families and thus could only sit on the sidelines. When anyone could do social work, the members lost an advocate invested with the professional and institutional authority to speak on their behalf from outside the medical perspective.

If social work is defined as a set of tasks, it may sometimes be the case that other kinds of workers can do what needs to be done. However, when social work is taken up by other providers, it is not only the work that gets reordered but the arsenal of solutions (Hughes 1970). When problems that might have appeared in social work appeared in the clinic, the geography of sense-making was altered. When these problems were taken up by workers not imbued with credentialed authority, members might have lost an advocate with enough institutional power to "speak back" to medical authority. At the Grove, the contraction of social work constrained not only the aspirations of social workers but also the care that members received.

The inner workings of the Grove were particular to this time, this place, and these people. Yet the devalued status of social work in relation to medical work is not a feature unique to the Grove. Nor are the interrelated challenges of disease, racism, and poverty unique to the Grove's members. In writing this account, one of my aims is to demonstrate how the expanded category of clinic problems is inextricably linked to the misrecognition of social inequality. Social inequality is a feature of most known human societies. Sociologists have long grappled with explaining its reproduction. Certainly, the naked exercise of state power can keep citizens from fomenting change. However, the sociologist Pierre Bourdieu (1991) observed that inequality is most effectively reproduced through symbolic power rather than hard power. Symbolic power can be summarized as "the ability to make appear as natural, inevitable, and thus apolitical that which is a product of historical struggle" (Loveman 2005, 1655). When the workings of power are hidden, resistance is not only avoided; it cannot even be cognitively conceived. There appears to be no power at work to resist. Bourdieu defined the act of obscuring power relations as misrecognition. Misrecognition creates legitimacy for the existing social order by concealing power relations and allowing them to go unchallenged (Bourdieu 1990; James 2015). In his own work, Bourdieu located processes of misrecognition in the social institution of education. I argue that misrecognition is also powerfully at work in the social institution of medicine.

The solution of the NP creates the appearance that what is amiss is our economic accounting. Nurse practitioners may not be a panacea, but they are a reasonable approach to rebalancing the health care equation of supply, demand, and cost. What is obscured in this framing of the solution is the source of the problem. Privatization of health care and the retrenchment of the welfare state is the primary diagnosis for what ails the Grove's members. The problems of poverty are not just problems that patients bring; they are also problems that the state has failed to address in other realms. For many of the Grove's members, the triage their NPs performed from inside the clinic was a lifeline. But lifelines are only needed when one is drowning. While the threat of being swallowed whole by social inequality can be ameliorated in the clinic, addressing the problems of inequality from within a clinic encounter removes it from other realms of problem-solving.

When NPs reconstitute a broad array of problems as clinic problems, they are pressed into the service of performing invisible work for their employer, but they are also part of a set of processes that render invisible the inaction of the state. The individualized interventions that come out of the clinic cannot address the systemic features of social inequality. It is not, however, my intention to argue that social work is the rightful professional home for such problems. Just as nursing is not a purposeful agent of misrecognition, social work cannot be the professional agent of its unraveling. The notion that inequality can be solved through the application of professional expertise itself obscures the workings of power.

It is true that social work has a unique professional history of calling attention to the structural conditions of inequality (Ehrenreich 1985). The beginnings of professional social work emerged from the settlement house movement of the early twentieth century. In contrast to traditional forms of charity or philanthropy, settlement workers lived within the communities they wished to help, providing direct services, organizing social events, and fighting alongside residents for social change (Koerin 2003). Settlement workers became a part of the community rather than just helpful benefactors. When the Grove's social workers link their profession with client empowerment, the settlement house tradition is one part of their history that they are in conversation with.

Yet the settlement house movement inspired not only the emerging profession of social work but also the nascent one of nursing. The nurses Lillian Wald and Mary Brewster founded the famous Henry Street Nurses' settlement in New York because they believed that bringing nursing out into the community and helping people as they worked to help themselves was not just something well-meaning individuals did, it was something that nurses should do (Wald 1902, 1915). The Henry Street Settlement became the birthplace of the vibrant tradition of public health nursing.

This common history illustrates that it may be less helpful to adjudicate the relative merits of two professional toolkits than it is to note that the settlement house tradition was a social and political movement, not a professional one. Settlement workers labored to reveal and address the structural causes of inequality, even as they worked pragmatically to ameliorate the conditions of poverty. The purview of social justice may not reside comfortably in the jurisdiction of any occupational group whose work must be justified by a nation-state that has fully embraced neoliberalism. A central tenet of neoliberalism is the inherent desirability of transferring the work of governments to the private market (Centeno and Cohen 2012). The US has become an exemplar of a privatized welfare state, where public resources are redistributed through private rather than public channels. The NP has become, in effect, a privatized, professional solution to social inequality, while social workers are largely left to fill out paperwork that disciplines and polices client access to the few social services that remain (Lipsky 1980; Schram and Silverman 2012; Smith and Lipsky 2009).

Conclusion

We are living through a crisis of care. In 2014, one in seven Americans was over the age of sixty-five. By 2060, that ratio will be closer to one in four (Colby and Ortman 2015). While medical advances have made old age healthier, it remains a part of the life course that requires increased support. The efficacy of preventive and curative strategies has had an independent hand in reshaping patient needs. Chronic conditions have increasingly replaced the acute in terms of mortality and disease burden (Gaziano 2010; Olshansky and Ault 1986; Omran 1971, 1977). We have never been more in need of care-centric practices.

The care crisis, however, is not exactly the one that NPs were created to solve. Although there are differences of opinion about what NPs should do, there has been little disagreement about what they are for: to help patients and health care organizations deal with physician scarcity. The NP is purported to be an economical and flexible stand-in, needed to address the dearth of physicians in an ever-expanding number of places. In this book, I have focused on their original proving ground of primary care, yet NPs are increasingly being used in a diversity of settings, from nursing homes to the acute care hospital. Moreover, the NP is just one example of nursing stepping into the breach left by physicians. Certified nurse midwives are taking on the work of obstetricians by providing prenatal care and attending vaginal births. Certified nurse anesthetists, one of nursing's oldest advance practice specialties, are helping hospitals deal with the scarcity and expense of anesthesiologists. It seems that almost anywhere physician labor is of concern, nurses are stepping in to ease the burdens of organizations and the patients they serve.

Throughout the health care system, nurses of all kinds are being rhetorically deployed as physician substitutes. It behooves us, however, to look underneath what people say and to look more closely at what they do. The rubric of substitution allows us to neatly fit the NP into equations of cost and personnel, but the calculus of social life is rarely that simple. I began my own investigations by trying to understand what the educators of NPs do to remake RNs into autonomous medical providers. I found that nursing educators were not attempting to create physician substitutes; they were engaged in the radical proposition that nurses can be skilled, independent providers without being like physicians. In the classrooms of Stanton Nursing School, students were provided with a history, orientation, and set of skills that served to distinguish the work of NPs from that of physicians, even as they borrowed from the physician's traditional toolkit of diagnostic medicine (Trotter 2019). At the Grove, this narrative construction of nursing difference had real-world consequences. The Grove's NPs were univocal in the belief that nurses possessed a distinct set of strategies that they brought to the medical encounter. Their attention to nursing's approach manifested in a stance of professional openness. They all, in their own ways, found themselves "doing what nurses do" by marshaling clinical, professional, and organizational resources to address a broad set of patient problems. The space that had been set aside for medical work soon became the site of clinic work.

In this book, however, I have endeavored to illustrate not just what NPs do, but what others do with them. The Grove ostensibly hired its NPs for their medical expertise, but in practice, it deployed them as much more than substitute physicians. In addition to the mandates of medical work, the Grove held its NPs uniquely responsible for care coordination. On the ground, this responsibility manifested as an obligation to "put out fires" for members and the organization rather than as an affirmative embodiment of NP authority. The physicians in particular withheld acknowledgment of NP expertise and therefore independent authority in patient care. Given the vocal antagonism of the AMA, this is not surprising. The physicians, however, were not the only ones. The Grove's administrators, some of whom were nurses, either failed to see the breadth of NP work, or failed to recognize that work as important to patient outcomes.

The NPs' performance of organizational care work had become the cornerstone of the Grove's goal of comprehensive care provision. Yet it was equally clear that the work and expertise required to meet this goal were largely unacknowledged. The logic of interchangeability that has legitimated the expansion of nursing independence has simultaneously rendered invisible the material work that nurses perform. According to the paperwork from payers, the balance sheets of organizations, and the mental logics of administrators, only medical work counts, even when more than medical work is expected. Nurse practitioners are normally studied to see how well they meet the gold standard of physician practice. But on the ground, NPs are often held to a higher standard than physicians—asked to medically attend to patients while also attending to the economic and coordination problems of patients and their employers.

Arlene Kaplan Daniels (1987) observed that much of the invisible work that women perform could be described as the labor of making social institutions work. In the domestic sphere, the invisible work of women holds families together (DeVault 1994; Oakley 2018). In the public sphere, the invisible work of women holds communities together through their unpaid work in schools as well as civic and cultural organizations (Daniels 1987, 1988). Scholars studying the paid labor market have shown how women, particularly women of color, make the economics of caregiving work (Diamond 1992; Glenn 1992; Stacey 2011). As physicians hold fast to protecting their status as professionals, it is nurses who are often left with the invisible work of holding health care together. They are doing so not just by performing medical work, but by performing care work for patients and organizations.

Although created as a solution to physician scarcity, the NP is just as often working on the front lines of our crisis in care. Nurse practitioners' work often goes unrecognized, but their performance of it has the potential to transform how patients experience the health care encounter. Some have quietly begun to question the logic of reimbursing NPs' labor at a lower rate than that of physicians. Their clinical responsibilities are not always the same, but when they are, one wonders whether paying NPs less violates the principle of equal pay for equal work. The answer to this question will be worked out in political rather than scholarly realms. But I will end with the observation that NPs are often *not* doing the same work as physicians. I make no claims that they are necessarily providing better care than physicians, but it is almost certainly more than medicine. In this account, my aim is not only to reveal the hidden work of yet another location of feminized labor but also to shine a light on the central importance of that work for patients.

A Gendered Solution

That more is expected of the NPs is not, I argue, limited to the particularities of the Grove. It is a reality produced by the gendered constraints faced by nursing as well as the gendered professional privilege held by medicine. The scarcity and unequal distribution of physicians has never been just a question of economics;

it is a question of power. To many readers, the high status of the US physician may appear to be a given. Medicine's prestige is something one assumes it has earned through the acquisition of expert knowledge. History, however, shows us that physicians' status was not bestowed; it was won. In his sweeping historical analysis, Paul Starr describes the political and cultural strategies through which US physicians transformed themselves from a powerless collection of low-status individuals into a powerful profession with authority over an increasing proportion of social life (Starr 1984). In the contemporary moment, physician dominance has undoubtedly taken a beating; yet physicians have managed to hang on to many of the perquisites of professional status, including autonomy. Professional medicine has been able to wield that autonomy to largely protect physician work from the influence of health care organizations and the state, even as individual physicians find themselves increasingly working within organizations and remunerated by state payers.

By contrast, nursing has never attained this level of power. Nursing has successfully expanded its domain of work and has significantly raised the status and pay of its denizens. Nonetheless, it has mostly labored in the shadow of medicine's authority. Nursing's inability to legitimately claim its own authority is one reason why scholars have dismissed it as an analytically minor actor in health care (Etzioni 1969; Freidson 1988a; F. E. Katz 1969). However, scholars who study the experience of women in the labor market have questioned a normative reading of occupational authority that erases the role of gender. These scholars have argued that female-dominated occupations have had to rely on different strategies from those adopted by male-dominated ones, because they do not have the same access to formal centers of power (Bourgeault 2006; Witz 1990, 1992). Without access to foundations, the higher education system, and political networks, women have historically relied more heavily on gendered appeals of moral authority. The audience to whom these appeals are made consists of state and organizational actors. As an occupation populated primarily by women, nursing's access to organizational and state support has largely been achieved through its responsiveness to employer and state concerns.

It is unlikely that NPs would have come into existence through arguments of skill alone. The doors of the exam room were opened because someone was in need. Patients needed providers; health care organizations needed medical personnel; the state needed to meet its moral obligation to care for its citizens while balancing the rising costs of care. Contrary to the prevailing narrative of substitution, I argue that NPs were called into being precisely because they were not physicians. Legitimated by professional authority, physicians could ignore the problems of health care organizations and the state. Nursing's reliance on moral authority has called them to be responsive to these neglected clients.

Nursing has a long history of doing so, from Nightingale in the late nineteenth century to public health nursing in the early twentieth century (D'Antonio 2017; Reverby 1987a). The NP is the newest addition in a long line of nursing solutions intended to address organizational and social ills as well as bodily ones.

There may, however, be unrecognized consequences arising from the shape of this solution. There is a robust literature that investigates the processes through which social problems are constructed. Problems themselves are not objective or quantitatively defined but are made through the rhetorical claims and political actions of concerned groups and individuals (Best 2017; Blumer 1971; Spector and Kitsuse 2017). Someone has to make the case that our attention and resources should go here rather than there. A parallel process that has received somewhat less scholarly attention is the construction and framing of solutions. Solutions are no more objectively defined than the problems that precede them. Moreover, the solution put forward often serves to reshape our understanding of the problem.

The NP is a reasonable solution to the problem of physician scarcity. I argue, however, that a focus on numbers of workers is a misrecognition of the real problem at hand. The crisis of care is not just about changing demography. Nor is it just about producing enough workers or figuring out the right calculus to pay for them. This crisis is, above all, a reflection of our changing view of what kinds of problems are amenable to public policy. When faced with the problems of physician scarcity and rising costs, the state had any number of choices at its disposal. It could have declared health care a public good and matched the weight of its financial investment with a more cohesive health care policy. When faced with entrenched health disparities along the lines of socioeconomic status—problems that have increasingly been traced to social structure rather than poor individual choices—the state might have invested in social welfare policies to ameliorate the worst excesses of living in poverty. When faced with the documented racial inequalities that the women and men of the Grove faced throughout their lives, the state might have chosen to put resources into eradicating entrenched forms of discrimination. Instead, the state outsourced its moral obligations to the private ministrations of a profession. In the personage of the NP, nursing has stepped forward to solve a set of problems as a profession that the state has been unwilling to address through social policy. In this account, I endeavor to reveal the hidden work of NPs. Through doing so, I also hope I have shined a small light on the hidden inaction of the state.

There are many things that ethnographic evidence cannot do. One of those things is provide average portraits. I do not claim that the work these NPs did is exactly like the work of their peers inside other organizations. The Grove is a single case, and a strange one at that. It is not lost on me that the Grove's entire reason for being is predicated on its uniqueness as an organizational form. The ability these NPs had to reorder clinic work was almost certainly out of proportion to that of other practice locations. The overlap between the Grove's mission of comprehensive care and nursing's claims of expertise over patient management was also likely an amplification of how primary care unfolds elsewhere.

For the purposes of an ethnographer, however, this strangeness was useful. Strange cases provide an analytical lens through which one can see, as if through a magnifying glass, a set of social processes and cultural understandings that exist elsewhere in less prominent forms. The Grove was unique, but the understandings these providers and administrators used to negotiate their day-to-day work were not entirely a local creation. Social life may be constructed, but the tools we use to construct that life are shared. In attaining a magnified view of these shared understandings, it was helpful that the Grove was strange in known and systematic ways. The organization's explicit commitment to nursing expertise made it easier to see the relationship between nursing ideals and practice, while the presence of the social workers made it possible to see society's disinvestment in nonmedical renderings of social problems.

Equally consequential is the fact that the Grove, as aberrant as it was, was also a real health care organization that operated under a field-level set of conditions: the enduring presence of physicians, an insured patient population who had some element of choice in how they accessed health care, and the dictates of third-party payers. These conditions made it possible to trace connections between realities on the ground and a particular set of structural realities having to do with the shrinking welfare state, the rising needs of an aging society, and the depth of the policy vacuum that nursing has stepped into.

The depth of that vacuum cannot be understated. In the face of shrinking resources for social welfare programs, both community activists and state workers are contemplating using health care funding to pay for a range of social benefits from housing to nutrition (Abrams 2019). Any progress in providing the socially vulnerable with basic needs would seem to require little justification. But there are, perhaps, missed opportunities to recognize the solidity of social problems as real problems. The relocation of what could be considered social, political, or community concerns to the realm of the clinic may produce a payer, but there may be unintended consequences for turning all problems into clinic problems. The tools of medicine, no matter who wields them, allow for some interventions and not others.

There are unanswered questions that an analysis of the NP makes visible. These questions are about neither professional nor academic concerns. They are inherently political questions about how to conceive of local and national solutions to social inequality. I have no answers of my own, but I will end this account with an alternate vision of what kind of organization the Grove might have been. I will ground that vision not by looking toward an imagined future, but by looking at the documented past.

An Alternate Vision

"This used to be a nursing home." When people recounted the Grove's history, this was often how the telling began. The role of the nursing home in this story needs little explanation. Nursing homes are instantly recognizable as an institutional villain for whom no one cheers. That the Grove is literally inhabiting the space of a former nursing home is ironic. It is karmic. It is a very satisfying story to tell. But it's not the only story. From 1978 to 2002, the building that Forest Grove would eventually occupy was the home of the Nathaniel Turner Nursing Home (a pseudonym). At its inception, the Turner Home served a primarily African American population. And that was a point of pride. It was created to be a community institution, for and by black residents.

The community that birthed the Turner Home had a long history of institutional building. The black southern migrants who streamed into northern cities in the early part of the twentieth century swelled the demographic footprint of the African American community in ways that supported cultural and organizational growth, even under the constraints of segregation. By 1950, the city that would later support the Turner Home already sustained a network of black churches, small businesses, banks, and theaters. This rich institutional life was both an adaptive response to exclusion from white institutions and a positive choice for community building.

By 1970, however, the death knell of black institutions was resounding throughout northeastern and midwestern cities. State-enforced urban renewal destroyed the architectural fabric of black life as families and business were forced out through government-backed projects of "slum clearance," freeway construction, and real estate projects that benefited white businesses at the expense of existing black occupants (Massey and Denton 1993). The gains of the Civil Rights Movement had also made the promise of racial integration into at least a partial reality. As African Americans began to have access to previously white institutions, the practical need to maintain separate institutions waned.

It was in this historical moment that the Turner Home was conceived. Built from the ground up, the Turner Home cost 3.5 million dollars to construct. Its board members spent years securing financing from local and national banks, eventually receiving additional support from the state and from the federal government's housing and urban development fund. The facility was described as state-of-the-art with an eye toward efficiency; it was, in the words of the board president, an attempt to provide "the best [care] for the most." But the vision of its founders was about more than simply providing health care. Although explicitly a nursing home, the Turner Home had a larger, intergenerational vision of community uplift. In addition to nursing home services, the founders hoped that the Turner Home would provide short-term material assistance for older adults who lived in its community. The board of directors looked toward a future when the Turner Home might eventually incorporate educational training for young black men and women in the health professions. Their vision was of an institution that would serve a broad spectrum of interconnected community needs.

From its very beginnings, it was an ambitious project. Perhaps too ambitious. By the late 1970s, opening a black institution of this scale seemed almost anachronistic. But the needs of the community were hard to deny. Despite the rhetoric of integration, African Americans still experienced segregated fortunes in housing, education, and health care. The long shadow of racial discrimination had a particular influence on the care and treatment of older adults. By the 1970s, nursing home care had become an increasingly viable option as a result of the passage of Medicare and Medicaid legislation. This legislation slowly transformed a sector that had previously been funded by private monies into one increasingly funded by public monies.

Despite public funding, African Americans were less likely than white Americans to access this kind of care. This was true in the 1970s and it remains true today. This racial difference has been long noted, but its explanation is not straightforward (Akamigbo and Wolinsky 2007; Cagney and Agree 1999; Smith et al. 2007; Thomeer, Mudrazija, and Angel 2015; Wallace et al. 1998). It has become almost a truism in health policy circles to point to cultural differences between white and black Americans. African Americans, scholars opine, think differently about family. But direct and structural discrimination bear at least as much consideration as love of family. Hospitals that wanted to receive Medicare and Medicaid reimbursements were forced to abide by the 1964 Civil Rights Act and desegregate their wards. However, it would be many more decades before federal funding was a significant portion of what was still a relatively small nursing home industry. Most white-only nursing homes relied on private-pay residents; attempts to open their doors to African Americans would have driven away their customers (Smith 1990). The federal government was also reluctant to enforce integration in spaces considered intimate or private, such as residential facilities (Smith 1990). There is also the much more straightforward reality of racial bias in nursing home admissions (Falcone and Broyles 1994; Institute of Medicine 1981). African Americans who found they needed nursing home care often struggled to find it.

In this context, the Turner Home was to be a place where black elders could receive the kind of care they were denied elsewhere. As the physical embodiment of an older vision of community and self-help, the Nathaniel Turner Nursing Home was to be an exemplar of what black institutions could still be. There was so much promise at its inauguration. One might be inclined to hope that it did at least some of what it set out to do—until the moment when we know that it did not. In 1998, investigations of the Turner Home found several deficiencies in patient care. The Turner Home was part of a growing number of nursing homes that were found wanting in quality. While this could be blamed in part on unscrupulous operators, there were also larger changes in the industry that challenged the entire sector. The "gold rush" of federal money into nursing home care created demand, but it also increased the cost. With federal money came federal regulation—the expense of which pushed many smaller nursing homes out of the market. For example, compliance with federal fire and safety codes was impossible for mom-and-pop facilities operating out of converted residential homes (Hawes and Phillips 1986).

As a response to legal action by the federal government and the challenges of running a smaller facility, the Turner Home permanently closed its doors in 2002. The building was emptied of residents and would stand vacant for the next four years. Eventually, the property went into foreclosure. City tax records contain a photograph that documents the building's fate: an empty parking lot, letters missing from the nursing home's sign, and windows that had been boarded up in defeat. The building that cost 3.5 million to build in the 1970s was bought by a developer for less than half a million in 2003.

It is unclear exactly when the dream of a community institution died. But perhaps when Stanton investigated the property in 2005, it recognized something of that original spirit. But Stanton had a somewhat different vision of what kind of institution the Grove would be. Like the Turner Home before it, the Grove served an almost exclusively African American population. But it was not to be a black institution. It was to be a nursing institution. As a practice of Stanton School of Nursing, its mission was not about racial uplift but about caring for the medically underserved. Stanton hoped it could still be a place to experience community. However, this vision of community formation was confined to the organizational apparatus of a health care organization.

Despite the best of intentions, the Grove sometimes struggled to make itself part of the community in ways that went beyond service provision. NP Francesca made this point to me in one of our interviews. She noted that the Grove "had the potential to be an ideal community practice, although it's not there yet." She provided an example of the kind of community partnership that would move the Grove closer to this ideal. "What if we opened a small training program here for community members who wanted to learn to be nursing assistants so that they could go out and make money? They could come here; we could teach them; they could do their practicum right here with our members. . . . I've brought this up a couple times and haven't gotten any place. But it's like, how great could that be?"

SW Yvonne also questioned the impermeability of the walls that seemed to have grown between the Grove and the community outside. In one of our conversations, she noted that the Grove was so keen on "re-creating community" within the center that it seemed to have forgotten that members were already part of communities. She wondered what would happen if the Grove moved beyond medical definitions of therapeutic socialization and instead worked in tandem with neighborhood organizations to strengthen the bonds of community. The mutual visions of Francesca and Yvonne, an NP and a social worker, may seem idealistically utopian. But perhaps it would be easier to imagine these visions in a different terrain. The alternatives they imagined may be impossible for a health care organization, but they might not be inconceivable for a community organization—one that saw its role as an agent of change rather than as a provider of services.

Appendix

TABLE 1 Demographic and salary data for employed registered nurses, nurse practitioners, and physicians and surgeons in the US, 2017

	REGISTERED NURSES	NURSE PRACTITIONERS	PHYSICIANS AND SURGEONS
Number	2,906,840	166,280	355,460
Median age	43.5	44.7	41.0
% female	89.9	92.2	40.0
% African American	12.3	10.6	8.2
% white	76.7	84.7	72.0
% Hispanic (any race)	6.9	3.4	6.8
% Asian	8.7	4.0	18.1
Mean salary	$73,550	$107,480	$211,390

Source: Data compiled from the Bureau of Labor Statistics, Current Population Survey, 2017, https://www.bls.gov/cps/.

TABLE 2 Clinical careers in nursing

	MOST COMMON ENTRY TO PRACTICE	ALTERNATE ENTRY TO PRACTICE	LEGACY ENTRY TO PRACTICE
Registered nurse (RN)	Bachelor's of science in nursing (BSN)	Associate's degree in nursing (ADN)[b]	Diploma certificate[d]
Nurse practitioner (NP)	Master's of science in nursing (MSN)[a]	Doctorate of nursing practice (DNP)[c]	
Certified nurse midwife (CNM)	Master's of science in nursing (MSN)[a]	Doctorate of nursing practice (DNP)[c]	
Clinical nurse specialist (CNS)	Master's of science in nursing (MSN)[a]	Doctorate of nursing practice (DNP)[c]	
Certified registered nurse anesthetist (CRNA)	Master's of science in nursing (MSN)[a]	Doctorate of nursing practice (DNP)[c]	

[a] NP, CNM, CNS, and CRNA credentialing requires an RN license.

[b] The ADN is typically completed in two to three years at a community college.

[c] The DNP is promoted by nursing advocates but is still uncommon among practicing NPs, CNMs, CNSs, and CRNAs.

[d] Diploma training is typically completed in two to three years within a hospital. This option is increasingly rare today.

Notes

INTRODUCTION

1. Throughout the book, I have chosen to refer to NPs and RNs as if they belong to mutually exclusive groups. This choice, however, is an inaccurate reflection of how credentialing in nursing works. Nursing uses an additive model; one begins with an RN license and then may obtain additional licenses through further education (see table 2 in the appendix). However, additional certifications do not "erase" the previous one. As a consequence, the broader group of RNs includes nurses with a range of educational preparations and responsibilities. Some RNs practice with a community college associate's degree. Others, like the NP, have obtained a master's degree in order to practice with a higher level of autonomy. The difficulty for the writer is that there is no tidy label that means "an RN without an advanced degree." Therefore, I have chosen to sacrifice accuracy for intelligibility. When referring to the Grove's nurses, I use "RN" to describe registered nurses who are not also NPs.

2. All names are pseudonyms. In the case of patient descriptions, some identifying information has been changed or obscured. Some medical profiles are composites of several patients. The decision to change descriptive details does carry a risk of affecting the analysis. In the appendix to the second edition of *Forgive and Remember*, Charles Bosk reflected on his decision to change the gender of a female surgical resident in order to mask her identity: "I have no doubt that changing genders theoretically impoverished my discussion of the moral order of surgical training. I also have no doubt that under the circumstances, I had little choice but to switch Jones' gender" (2011, 211). In describing medical information about patients, I also have little choice. However, as this book is primarily an account of workers rather than patients, I am reasonably confident that these changes do not significantly affect the analysis that follows. There are places where I have obscured staff positions, but I have done so through omission rather than fictionalizing or changing details. The reader, then, can make an informed decision about how much the lack of detail may affect the reported findings.

3. There is an entrenched hierarchy in health care that is reproduced through symbolic as well as material means. Titles are an enduring symbolic distinction that separate medicine from every other occupation. Physicians are given the title of "Doctor" as an acknowledgement of their credentialing achievement. There is no analogous title to acknowledge the achievement of becoming a nurse or social worker, regardless of educational credentials. At the Grove, physicians were referred to as Dr. Morgan and Dr. Michaels. Everyone else, including the NPs, were referred to by their first names. In this account, I have remained true to the words chosen by the people at the Grove when they spoke to and about one another. However, when using my own words, I have chosen, in my own small way, to resist reproducing this hierarchy. As each clinician makes a first appearance within a chapter, I have used either a traditional or a new title, such as "Dr. Christine Morgan" or "NP Michelle." In subsequent mentions, I refer to all clinicians by their first names. I have included the last names of physicians at first mention (and omitted the last names of other staff) so that my own naming convention is in concordance with, if not the same as, those used inside the Grove.

4. In reality, many home care aides make the decision to step in when clients need such assistance (Stacey 2011). They choose to "act like family" (or feel pressured by their

employers) to do what needs to be done despite its illegality. However, aides cannot be asked to do so by the agencies that employ them; nor could a health care provider write a plan of care that requests an aide to do so.

5. There is a constantly shifting landscape of regulations that depends on state as well as practice location. In institutional settings, a much broader range of workers can often dispense medication under the supervision of an RN or physician. In the community setting, some states are beginning to allow home care aides to do so in particular circumstances. However, in the state where Ms. Payne resided, the choices were limited to an RN or physician.

6. Medicaid eligibility requirements are set at the state level and vary considerably from state to state. In particular, after the passage of the Affordable Care Act, many states chose to expand Medicaid access as a way of providing affordable insurance to more adults.

7. For example, some scholars separate out nurturant care work from non-nurturant care work in order to acknowledge the difference between, for example, the interactive work of a nurse and the less interactive work of a janitor (Duffy 2005).

1. NURSING'S EXPERTISE

1. Although nursing was to be a separate, woman's profession, its doors were not open to every woman. For Nightingale and her followers in the US, the doorway to nursing was both classed and raced. Although she was suspicious of the upper-class "ladies" who desired to volunteer as nurses, Nightingale's equation of moral character with class created a clear preference for middle-class over working-class women for leadership roles (Holton 1984). In a letter in which she delivered advice on creating hospitals in colonial India, she wrote, "Wherever there is more than one female Nurse [sic] there must be one woman in the position of Matron, and she must, of course, be an [sic] European" (Nightingale 1865, 10). A similar prejudice developed in the US. In their desire to rescue nursing from the province of servants, the first US nursing schools explicitly barred women already working in domestic service. Some even took steps to bar white women from ethnic groups associated with domestic service (Reverby 1987a). The options for black women were even more severely restricted. They were segregated into inferior training programs, excluded from professional nursing organizations, and prohibited from most nursing positions until the 1970s (Hine 1989).

2. Even the Grove could not entirely escape the dominant assumption of physician leadership. A few months into my fieldwork, the Grove's administration was surprised to discover that under their program regulations, NPs were not allowed to be the provider of record. Although they were able to rectify this problem by submitting a formal waiver request, it was telling that the Grove had to petition the federal government, not for NPs to do the work—their NPs were already practicing in accordance with state law—but merely to do so under their own names.

2. FROM MEDICAL WORK TO CLINIC WORK

1. A notable exception is the work of Sue Fisher (1995). She has published one of the only in-depth, qualitative studies that attempts to describe and account for differences between NPs and physicians in the health care encounter.

3. ORGANIZATIONAL CARE WORK

1. See table 1 in the appendix for salary and demographic data of RNs, NPs, and physicians and surgeons.

4. NEW BOUNDARIES, NEW RELATIONSHIPS

1. The role and identity of the clinical nurse specialist (CNS) is difficult to define, primarily because employers have remained ambivalent about the role. Clinical nurse

specialists were created at a time when most working nurses lacked a college degree. As one of the first graduate-trained nurses, the CNS was originally created to serve as "the expert nurse" in the hospital setting, providing staff education and directing care for a ward or patient population. In an unfortunate twist of fate, the creation of the NP largely eclipsed the CNS. Today, many hospitals have no role that is specific to the CNS. Many CNSs find themselves competing for hospital jobs with nurses of a variety of educational backgrounds. Moreover, their traditional inability to independently provide and bill for services makes them a hard sell for outpatient settings that cannot bundle costs. As a result, CNSs have started to press for prescriptive authority and practice independence so they can treat individual patients as NPs already do—a strategy which only makes their specific expertise even harder to pin down for employers and the general public.

2. The case of nursing credentialing is an example of how nursing's professionalizing aims have been tempered by the labor needs of hospitals—the primary employers of nurses. Changing industry standards have pressured hospitals to move toward requiring BSNs from their nursing staff. However, in no state is any hospital legally barred from hiring associate's-trained RNs. It is not considered best practice, but hospitals can and do employ them. However, there is some movement on that front. In 2018, New York became the first state to pass legislation requiring that new nurses earn a bachelor's degree within ten years of their initial licensure. But even this groundbreaking legislation applies only to newly licensed nurses and not to those already in practice.

5. GAINING STATUS, LOSING GROUND

1. Anecdotally, there are some physicians who believe that NPs take longer to see patients because they are less skilled. I cannot evaluate that assessment (neither, of course, have they). I can, however, offer these words from NP Michelle: "Each [enrollment] takes two hours to do and I feel confident that I'm not just a person that's just taking longer than other people because when we went to [a conference of similar organizations], I asked the medical director [in Saint Louis] who does the assessments there. She said, 'Yeah, it takes me two hours.' That's a doctor, and it takes her two hours."

6. THE CONTRACTION OF SOCIAL WORK

1. I began my fieldwork as a volunteer without Institutional Review Board approval. Although no one told me I was forbidden to enter the clinic, I limited my exposure to protected health information until I had formal approval.

2. Prior to Yvonne's hiring, a copy of the Grove's organizational chart explicitly did not include the position of social work supervisor. By contrast, other unoccupied positions had vacant placeholders.

3. In a literal sense, the Grove did go without a director of nursing until NP Stephen's arrival. However, in a previous version of the organizational chart, the NPs answered to the chief operating officer, a position occupied by a nurse. This was no accident. Nursing has fought long and hard to be self-governed. It is rare that another profession is allowed to supervise nursing work.

7. THE MISRECOGNITION OF SOCIAL PROBLEMS

1. During most of my fieldwork, the organization was neither hiring nor employing case workers to assist the social work department. This position was phased out through attrition.

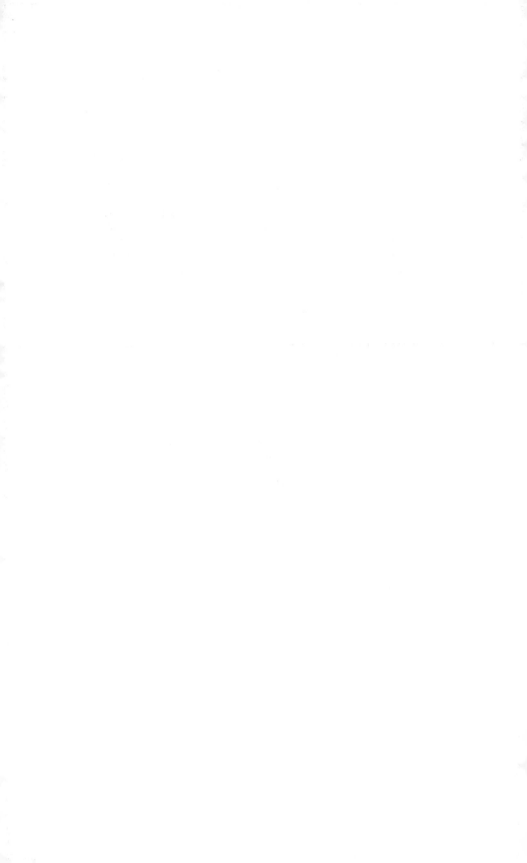

References

Abbott, Andrew. 1988. *The System of Professions: An Essay on the Division of Expert Labor.* Chicago: University of Chicago Press.

Abrams, Amanda. 2019. "Using Medicaid Dollars to Pay for Housing?" Shelterforce. Accessed July 28, 2019. https://shelterforce.org/2019/02/19/medicaid-dollars-for-housing/.

Adler, Nancy E., and Katherine Newman. 2002. "Socioeconomic Disparities in Health: Pathways and Policies." *Health Affairs* 21 (2): 60–76. https://doi.org/10.1377/hlthaff.21.2.60.

Agency for Healthcare Research and Quality. 2012. "Primary Care Workforce Facts and Stats." US Department of Health and Human Services. http://www.ahrq.gov/research/findings/factsheets/primary/pcworkforce/index.html.

Aiken, Linda H. 2014. "Baccalaureate Nurses and Hospital Outcomes: More Evidence." *Medical Care* 52 (10): 861–63. https://doi.org/10.1097/MLR.0000000000000222.

Aiken, Linda H., Sean P. Clarke, Douglas M. Sloane, Julie Sochalski, and Jeffrey H. Silber. 2002. "Hospital Nurse Staffing and Patient Mortality, Nurse Burnout, and Job Dissatisfaction." *JAMA: The Journal of the American Medical Association* 288 (16): 1987–93. https://doi.org/10.1001/jama.288.16.1987.

Akamigbo, Adaeze B., and Fredric D. Wolinsky. 2007. "New Evidence of Racial Differences in Access and Their Effects on the Use of Nursing Homes among Older Adults." *Medical Care* 45 (7): 672–79. https://doi.org/10.1097/MLR.0b013e3180455677.

Allen, Davina. 1997. "The Nursing-Medical Boundary: A Negotiated Order?" *Sociology of Health & Illness* 19 (4): 498–520.

——. 2000. "Doing Occupational Demarcation: The 'Boundary-Work' of Nurse Managers in a District General Hospital." *Journal of Contemporary Ethnography* 29 (3): 326–56.

——. 2001. "Narrating Nursing Jurisdiction: 'Atrocity Stories' and 'Boundary-Work.'" *Symbolic Interaction* 24 (1): 75–103.

——. 2004. "Re-reading Nursing and Re-writing Practice: Towards an Empirically Based Reformulation of the Nursing Mandate." *Nursing Inquiry* 11 (4): 271–83. https://doi.org/10.1111/j.1440-1800.2004.00234.x.

——. 2014. "Re-conceptualising Holism in the Contemporary Nursing Mandate: From Individual to Organisational Relationships." *Social Science & Medicine* 119: 131–38.

American Association of Nurse Practitioners. 2018. "Nurse Practitioner State Practice Environment." Last modified December 20, 2018. https://www.aanp.org/advocacy/state/state-practice-environment.

——. 2019. *NP Fact Sheet.* American Association of Nurse Practitioners. https://storage.aanp.org/www/documents/Npfacts.pdf.

American Medical Association. 2005. "Limited Licensure Health Care Provider Training and Certification Standards." AMA House of Delegates Resolution 814 (I-05).

———. 2017. *The AMA 2016 Annual Report*. American Medical Association. https://www.ama-assn.org/about-us/ama-annual-report.

American Nurses' Association. 1965. "American Nurses' Association's First Position on Education for Nursing." *American Journal of Nursing* 65 (12): 106–11.

Anspach, Renee R. 1997. *Deciding Who Lives: Fateful Choices in the Intensive-Care Nursery*. Berkeley: University of California Press.

Apesoa-Varano, Ester Carolina. 2007. "Educated Caring: The Emergence of Professional Identity among Nurses." *Qualitative Sociology* 30 (3): 249–74.

———. 2013. "Interprofessional Conflict and Repair: A Study of Boundary Work in the Hospital." *Sociological Perspectives* 56 (3): 327–49.

———. 2016. "Not Merely TLC: Nurses' Caring Revisited." *Qualitative Sociology* 39 (1): 27–47. https://doi.org/10.1007/s11133-015-9322-3.

Apesoa-Varano, Ester Carolina, and Charles S. Varano. 2014. *Conflicted Health Care: Professionalism and Caring in an Urban Hospital*. Nashville, TN: Vanderbilt University Press.

Aronson, Jane, and Kristin Smith. 2010. "Managing Restructured Social Services: Expanding the Social?" *British Journal of Social Work* 40 (2): 530–47. https://doi.org/10.1093/bjsw/bcp002.

Association of American Medical Colleges. 2017. "Table A-6: Age of Applicants to U.S. Medical Schools at Anticipated Matriculation by Sex and Race/Ethnicity, 2014–2015 through 2017–2018." In FACTS: Applicants, Matriculants, Enrollment, Graduates, MD-PhD, and Residency Applicants Data. Accessed December 20, 2018. https://www.aamc.org/data/facts/.

Auerbach, David I., Peter I. Buerhaus, and Douglas O. Staiger. 2014. "Registered Nurses Are Delaying Retirement, a Shift That Has Contributed to Recent Growth in the Nurse Workforce." *Health Affairs* 33 (8): 1474–80.

Baker, David P., Rachel Day, and Eduardo Salas. 2006. "Teamwork as an Essential Component of High-Reliability Organizations." *Health Services Research* 41 (4p2): 1576–98. https://doi.org/10.1111/j.1475-6773.2006.00566.x.

Barnes, Hilary. 2015. "Exploring the Factors That Influence Nurse Practitioner Role Transition." In "Health Policy." Special issue, *Journal for Nurse Practitioners* 11 (2): 178–83.

Becker, Howard S., Blanche Greer, Everett Cherrington Hughes, and Anselm Strauss. 1976. *Boys in White*. New Brunswick, NJ: Transaction.

Benner, Patricia, and Christine A. Tanner. 1987. "How Expert Nurses Use Intuition." *American Journal of Nursing* 87 (1): 23–34.

Best, Joel. 2017. *Images of Issues: Typifying Contemporary Social Problems*. New York: Routledge.

Blegen, Mary A., Colleen J. Goode, Shin Hye Park, Thomas Vaughn, and Joanne Spetz. 2013. "Baccalaureate Education in Nursing and Patient Outcomes." *Journal of Nursing Administration* 43 (2): 89–94. https://doi.org/10.1097/NNA.0b013e31827f2028.

Blumer, Herbert. 1954. "What Is Wrong With Social Theory?" *American Sociological Review* 19 (1): 3–10.

———. 1971. "Social Problems as Collective Behavior." *Social Problems* 18 (3): 298–306. https://doi.org/10.2307/799797.

Bosk, Charles L. 2011. *Forgive and Remember: Managing Medical Failure*. 2nd ed. Chicago: University of Chicago Press.

Bourdieu, Pierre. 1990. *The Logic of Practice*. Oxford: Polity Press.

———. 1991. *Language and Symbolic Power*. Cambridge, MA: Harvard University Press.

Bourgeault, Ivy Lynn. 2006. *Push!: The Struggle for Midwifery in Ontario*. Montreal: McGill-Queen's University Press.

Braveman, Paula A., Catherine Cubbin, Susan Egerter, Sekai Chideya, Kristen S. Marchi, Marilyn Metzler, and Samuel Posner. 2005. "Socioeconomic Status in Health Research: One Size Does Not Fit All." *JAMA: The Journal of the American Medical Association* 294 (22): 2879–88. https://doi.org/10.1001/jama.294.22.2879.

Braveman, Paula A., Susan Egerter, and David R. Williams. 2011. "The Social Determinants of Health: Coming of Age." *Annual Review of Public Health* 32 (1): 381–98. https://doi.org/10.1146/annurev-publhealth-031210-101218.

Brown, Marie-Annette, and Ellen Olshansky. 1998. "Becoming a Primary Care Nurse Practitioner: Challenges of the Initial Year of Practice." *Nurse Practitioner* 23 (7): 46–66.

Brush, Barbara L., and Elizabeth A. Capezuti. 1996. "Revisiting 'A Nurse for All Settings': The Nurse Practitioner Movement, 1965–1995." *Journal of the American Academy of Nurse Practitioners* 8 (1): 5–11. https://doi.org/10.1111/j.1745-7599.1996.tb01035.x.

Buerhaus, Peter, Jennifer Perloff, Sean Clarke, Monica O'Reilly-Jacob, Galina Zolotusky, and Catherine M. DesRoches. 2018. "Quality of Primary Care Provided to Medicare Beneficiaries by Nurse Practitioners and Physicians." *Medical Care* 56 (6): 484–90. https://doi.org/10.1097/MLR.0000000000000908.

Bureau of Labor Statistics. 2018a. "Occupational Outlook Handbook: Registered Nurses." U.S. Department of Labor. https://www.bls.gov/ooh/healthcare/registered-nurses.htm.

——. 2018b. "Occupational Outlook Handbook: Social Workers." U.S. Department of Labor. https://www.bls.gov/ooh/community-and-social-service/social-workers.htm.

Burwell, Sylvia Mathews. 2016. *Report to Congress: 2016 Actuarial Report on the Financial Outlook for Medicaid.* Centers for Medicare and Medicaid Services. https://www.medicaid.gov/medicaid/finance/downloads/medicaid-actuarial-report-2016.pdf.

Cagney, Kathleen A., and Emily M. Agree. 1999. "Racial Differences in Skilled Nursing Care and Home Health Use: The Mediating Effects of Family Structure and Social Class." *Journals of Gerontology Series B: Psychological Sciences and Social Sciences* 54 (4): S223–36. https://doi.org/10.1093/geronb/54B.4.S223.

Cassell, Joan. 1998. *The Woman in the Surgeon's Body.* Cambridge, MA: Harvard University Press.

Centeno, Miguel A., and Joseph N. Cohen. 2012. "The Arc of Neoliberalism." *Annual Review of Sociology* 38: 317–40. https://doi.org/10.1146/annurev-soc-081309-150235.

Chambliss, Daniel F. 1996. *Beyond Caring: Hospitals, Nurses, and the Social Organization of Ethics.* Chicago: University of Chicago Press.

Charles, Maria, and David Grusky. 2005. *Occupational Ghettos: The Worldwide Segregation of Women and Men.* Palo Alto, CA: Stanford University Press.

Colby, Sandra L., and Jennifer M. Ortman. 2015. *Projections of the Size and Composition of the U.S. Population: 2014 to 2060.* P25–1143. Current Population Reports. Washington, DC: U.S. Census Bureau.

Conrad, Peter. 1992. "Medicalization and Social Control." *Annual Review of Sociology* 18: 209–32. https://doi.org/10.1146/annurev.so.18.080192.001233.

——. 2005. "The Shifting Engines of Medicalization." *Journal of Health and Social Behavior* 46 (1): 3–14. https://doi.org/10.1177/002214650504600102.

——. 2007. *The Medicalization of Society: On the Transformation of Human Conditions into Treatable Disorders.* Baltimore: Johns Hopkins University Press.

Cornwell, Benjamin, Edward O. Laumann, and L. Philip Schumm. 2008. "The Social Connectedness of Older Adults: A National Profile." *American Sociological Review* 73 (2): 185–203.

Cornwell, Erin York, and Linda J. Waite. 2009a. "Social Disconnectedness, Perceived Isolation, and Health among Older Adults." *Journal of Health and Social Behavior* 50 (1): 31–48. https://doi.org/10.1177/002214650905000103.

——. 2009b. "Measuring Social Isolation among Older Adults Using Multiple Indicators from the NSHAP Study." *Journals of Gerontology Series B: Psychological Sciences and Social Sciences* 64 (1): i38–46. https://doi.org/10.1093/geronb/gbp037.

Cusson, Regina M., and Sally Nelson Strange. 2008. "Neonatal Nurse Practitioner Role Transition: The Process of Reattaining Expert Status." *Journal of Perinatal & Neonatal Nursing* 22 (4): 329–37.

Daniels, Arlene Kaplan. 1987. "Invisible Work." *Social Problems* 34 (5): 403–15. https://doi.org/10.2307/800538.

——. 1988. *Invisible Careers: Women Civic Leaders from the Volunteer World*. Chicago: University of Chicago Press.

D'Antonio, Patricia. 2017. *Nursing with a Message: Public Health Demonstration Projects in New York City*. New Brunswick, NJ: Rutgers University Press.

Davies, Karen. 2003. "The Body and Doing Gender: The Relations between Doctors and Nurses in Hospital Work." *Sociology of Health & Illness* 25 (7): 720–42. https://doi.org/10.1046/j.1467-9566.2003.00367.x.

DesRoches, Catherine M., Sean Clarke, Jennifer Perloff, Monica O'Reilly-Jacob, and Peter Buerhaus. 2017. "The Quality of Primary Care Provided by Nurse Practitioners to Vulnerable Medicare Beneficiaries." *Nursing Outlook* 65 (6): 679–88. https://doi.org/10.1016/j.outlook.2017.06.007.

DeVault, Marjorie L. 1994. *Feeding the Family: The Social Organization of Caring as Gendered Work*. Chicago: University of Chicago Press.

——. 2014. "Mapping Invisible Work: Conceptual Tools for Social Justice Projects." *Sociological Forum* 29 (4): 775–90. https://doi.org/10.1111/socf.12119.

Diamond, Timothy. 1992. *Making Gray Gold: Narratives of Nursing Home Care*. Chicago: University of Chicago Press.

Diers, Donna, and Susan Molde. 1983. "Nurses in Primary Care: The New Gatekeepers?" *American Journal of Nursing* 83 (5): 742–45.

Dingwall, Robert, and Davina Allen. 2001. "The Implications of Healthcare Reforms for the Profession of Nursing." *Nursing Inquiry* 8 (2): 64–74. https://doi.org/10.1046/j.1440-1800.2001.00100.x.

Drolet, Brian C., Matthew Schwede, Kenneth D. Bishop, and Staci A. Fischer. 2013. "Compliance and Falsification of Duty Hours: Reports from Residents and Program Directors." *Journal of Graduate Medical Education* 5 (3): 368–73. https://doi.org/10.4300/JGME-D-12-00375.1.

Duffy, Mignon. 2005. "Reproducing Labor Inequalities: Challenges for Feminists Conceptualizing Care at the Intersections of Gender, Race, and Class." *Gender & Society* 19 (1): 66–82. https://doi.org/10.1177/0891243204269499.

Duffy, Mignon, Randy Albelda, and Clare Hammonds. 2013. "Counting Care Work: The Empirical and Policy Applications of Care Theory." *Social Problems* 60 (2): 145–67. https://doi.org/10.1525/sp.2013.60.2.145.

Ehrenreich, John H. 1985. *The Altruistic Imagination: A History of Social Work and Social Policy in the United States*. Ithaca, NY: Cornell University Press.

England, Paula. 1992. *Comparable Worth: Theories and Evidence*. New York: Aldine de Gruyter.

——. 2005. "Emerging Theories of Care Work." *Annual Review of Sociology* 31: 381–99. https://doi.org/10.1146/annurev.soc.31.041304.122317.

——. 2010. "The Gender Revolution: Uneven and Stalled." *Gender & Society* 24 (2): 149–66. https://doi.org/10.1177/0891243210361475.

England, Paula, Michelle Budig, and Nancy Folbre. 2002. "Wages of Virtue: The Relative Pay of Care Work." *Social Problems* 49 (4): 455–73.

England, Paula, and Nancy Folbre. 1999. "The Cost of Caring." *Annals of the American Academy of Political and Social Science* 561 (1): 39–51. https://doi.org/10.1177/000271629956100103.

Etzioni, Amitai. 1969. "Introduction." In *The Semi-professions and Their Organization: Teachers, Nurses, and Social Workers*, edited by Amitai Etzioni, i–xviii. New York: Free Press.

Evans, Lois K. 1996. "Knowing the Patient: The Route to Individualized Care." *Journal of Gerontological Nursing* 22 (3): 15–19. https://doi.org/10.3928/0098-9134-19960301-07.

Evers, Helen. 1982. "Professional Practice and Patient Care: Multidisciplinary Teamwork in Geriatric Wards." *Ageing & Society* 2 (1): 57–76.

Fabricant, Michael, Steve F. Burghardt, and Irwin Epstein. 2016. *The Welfare State Crisis and the Transformation of Social Service Work*. New York: Routledge. https://doi.org/10.4324/9781315289175.

Fairman, Julie. 2008. *Making Room in the Clinic: Nurse Practitioners and the Evolution of Modern Health Care*. New Brunswick, NJ: Rutgers University Press.

Fairman, Julie, and Joan E. Lynaugh. 2000. *Critical Care Nursing: A History*. Philadelphia: University of Pennsylvania Press.

Falcone, David, and Robert Broyles. 1994. "Access to Long-Term Care: Race as a Barrier." *Journal of Health Politics, Policy and Law* 19 (3): 583–95.

Finn, Rachael. 2008. "The Language of Teamwork: Reproducing Professional Divisions in the Operating Theatre." *Human Relations* 61 (1): 103–30. https://doi.org/10.1177/0018726707085947.

Finn, Rachael, Mark Learmonth, and Patrick Reedy. 2010. "Some Unintended Effects of Teamwork in Healthcare." *Social Science & Medicine* 70 (8): 1148–54. https://doi.org/10.1016/j.socscimed.2009.12.025.

Fisher, Sue. 1995. *Nursing Wounds*. New Brunswick, NJ: Rutgers University Press.

Fox, Renee. 1957. "Training for Uncertainty." In *The Student Physician: Introductory Studies in the Sociology of Medical Education*, edited by Robert K. Merton, George G. Reader, and Patricia Kendall, 207–41. Cambridge, MA: Harvard University Press for the Commonwealth Fund.

Frankel, Richard M. 1990. "Talking in Interviews: A Dispreference for Patient-Initiated Questions in Physician-Patient Encounters." In *Interaction Competence*, edited by George Psathas, 231–64. Washington, DC: University Press of America.

Freedman, Vicki A., and Brenda C. Spillman. 2014. "Disability and Care Needs among Older Americans." *Milbank Quarterly* 92 (3): 509–41. https://doi.org/10.1111/1468-0009.12076.

Freidson, Eliot. 1970. *Professional Dominance: The Social Structure of Medical Care*. Piscataway, NJ: Aldine de Gruyter.

——. 1988a. *Profession of Medicine: A Study of the Sociology of Applied Knowledge*. Chicago: University of Chicago Press.

——. 1988b. "The Medical Division of Labor." In *Profession of Medicine: A Study of the Sociology of Applied Knowledge*, 47–70. Chicago: University of Chicago Press.

——. 1988c. *Professional Powers: A Study of the Institutionalization of Formal Knowledge*. Chicago: University of Chicago Press.

Gaziano, J. Michael. 2010. "Fifth Phase of the Epidemiologic Transition: The Age of Obesity and Inactivity." *JAMA: The Journal of the American Medical Association* 303 (3): 275–76. https://doi.org/10.1001/jama.2009.2025.

Genworth. 2018. *2018 Cost of Care Survey: Summary of Findings.* Genworth Financial. https://pro.genworth.com/riiproweb/productinfo/pdf/131168.pdf.

Geronimus, Arline T. 1996. "Black/White Differences in the Relationship of Maternal Age to Birthweight: A Population-Based Test of the Weathering Hypothesis." *Social Science & Medicine* 42 (4): 589–97. https://doi.org/10.1016/0277-9536(95)00159-X.

Geronimus, Arline T., Margaret Hicken, Danya Keene, and John Bound. 2006. "'Weathering' and Age Patterns of Allostatic Load Scores among Blacks and Whites in the United States." *American Journal of Public Health* 96 (5): 826–33. https://doi.org/10.2105/AJPH.2004.060749.

Gieryn, Thomas F. 1983. "Boundary-Work and the Demarcation of Science from Nonscience: Strains and Interests in Professional Ideologies of Scientists." *American Sociological Review* 48 (6): 781–95. https://doi.org/10.2307/2095325.

Ginzberg, Lori D. 1992. *Women and the Work of Benevolence: Morality, Politics, and Class in the Nineteenth-Century United States.* New Haven, CT: Yale University Press.

Glenn, Evelyn Nakano. 1992. "From Servitude to Service Work: Historical Continuities in the Racial Division of Paid Reproductive Labor." *Signs* 18 (1): 1–43.

Goldsmith, Jeff. 1993. "Hospital/Physician Relationships: A Constraint to Health Reform." *Health Affairs* 12 (3): 160–69. https://doi.org/10.1377/hlthaff.12.3.160.

Gordon, Suzanne, and Sioban Nelson. 2006. "Moving beyond the Virtue Script: Creating a Knowledge Based Identity for Nurses." In *The Complexities of Care: Nursing Reconsidered*, edited by Sioban Nelson and Suzanne Gordon, 13–29. Ithaca, NY: Cornell University Press.

Granfield, Robert. 1992. *Making Elite Lawyers: Visions of Law at Harvard and Beyond.* New York: Routledge.

Hafferty, Frederick W., and Ronald Franks. 1994. "The Hidden Curriculum, Ethics Teaching, and the Structure of Medical Education." *Academic Medicine: Journal of the Association of American Medical Colleges* 69 (11): 861–71.

Hawes, Catherine, and Charles D. Phillips. 1986. "The Changing Structure of the Nursing Home Industry and the Impact of Ownership on Quality, Cost, and Access." In *For-Profit Enterprise in Health Care*, edited by Bradford H. Gray. Washington, DC: National Academies Press. http://www.ncbi.nlm.nih.gov/books/NBK217907/.

Health Resource and Services Administration. 2014. *Highlights from the 2012 National Sample Survey of Nurse Practitioners.* Rockville, MD: US Department of Health and Human Services. https://bhw.hrsa.gov/sites/default/files/bhw/nchwa/npsurveyhighlights.pdf.

Heitz, Laura J., Susan H. Steiner, and Mary E. Burman. 2004. "RN to FNP: A Qualitative Study of Role Transition." *Journal of Nursing Education* 43 (9): 416–20.

Hill, Laura A., and Jo-Ann V. Sawatzky. 2011. "Transitioning into the Nurse Practitioner Role through Mentorship." *Journal of Professional Nursing* 27 (3): 161–67.

Himmelstein, David U., and Steffie Woolhandler. 2016. "The Current and Projected Taxpayer Shares of US Health Costs." *American Journal of Public Health* 106 (3): 449–52. https://doi.org/10.2105/AJPH.2015.302997.

Hine, Darlene Clark. 1989. *Black Women in White: Racial Conflict and Cooperation in the Nursing Profession, 1890–1950.* Bloomington: Indiana University Press.

Hochschild, Arlie Russell. 1983. *The Managed Heart: The Commercialization of Human Feeling.* Berkeley: University of California Press.

Holton, Sandra. 1984. "Feminine Authority and Social Order: Florence Nightingale's Conception of Nursing and Health Care." *Social Analysis: The International Journal of Social and Cultural Practice* 15: 59–72.

Horrocks, Sue, Elizabeth Anderson, and Chris Salisbury. 2002. "Systematic Review of Whether Nurse Practitioners Working in Primary Care Can Provide Equivalent Care to Doctors." *BMJ* 324 (7341): 819–23. https://doi.org/10.1136/bmj.324. 7341.819.

Hughes, Everett Cherrington. 1970. "The Humble and the Proud: The Comparative Study of Occupations." *Sociological Quarterly* 11 (2): 147–56. https://doi. org/10.1111/j.1533-8525.1970.tb01440.x.

——. 1981. *Men and Their Work*. Westport, CT: Greenwood Press.

Huguet, Nathalie, Mark S. Kaplan, and David Feeny. 2008. "Socioeconomic Status and Health-Related Quality of Life among Elderly People: Results from the Joint Canada/United States Survey of Health." *Social Science & Medicine* 66 (4): 803–10. https://doi.org/10.1016/j.socscimed.2007.11.011.

Institute of Medicine. 1981. *Health Care in a Context of Civil Rights*. Washington, DC: National Academy Press. https://doi.org/10.17226/18680.

——. 2001. *Crossing the Quality Chasm: A New Health System for the 21st Century*. Washington, DC: National Academies Press. https://doi.org/10.17226/10027.

James, David. 2015. "How Bourdieu Bites Back: Recognising Misrecognition in Education and Educational Research." *Cambridge Journal of Education* 45 (1): 97–112. https://doi.org/10.1080/0305764X.2014.987644.

Katz, Fred E. 1969. "Nurses." In *The Semi-professions and Their Organization: Teachers, Nurses, and Social Workers*, edited by Amitai Etzioni, 54–81. New York: Free Press.

Katz, Jay. 1984. *The Silent World of Doctor and Patient*. New York: Free Press.

Kellogg, Katherine C. 2011. *Challenging Operations: Medical Reform and Resistance in Surgery*. Chicago: University of Chicago Press.

Khan, Shamus. 2012. "The Sociology of Elites." *Annual Review of Sociology* 38: 361–77.

Koerin, Beverly. 2003. "The Settlement House Tradition: Current Trends and Future Concerns." *Journal of Sociology and Social Welfare* 30: 53–68.

Krause, Neal, Jason T. Newsom, and Karen S. Rook. 2008. "Financial Strain, Negative Social Interaction, and Self-Rated Health: Evidence from Two United States Nationwide Longitudinal Surveys." *Ageing & Society* 28 (7): 1001–23. https:// doi.org/10.1017/S0144686X0800740X.

Kunzel, Regina G. 1995. *Fallen Women, Problem Girls*. New Haven, CT: Yale University Press.

Landrigan, Christopher P., Laura K. Barger, Brian E. Cade, Najib T. Ayas, and Charles A. Czeisler. 2006. "Interns' Compliance with Accreditation Council for Graduate Medical Education Work-Hour Limits." *JAMA: The Journal of the American Medical Association* 296 (9): 1063–70. https://doi.org/10.1001/jama.296.9.1063.

Landsperger, Janna S., Matthew W. Semler, Li Wang, Daniel W. Byrne, and Arthur P. Wheeler. 2016. "Outcomes of Nurse Practitioner-Delivered Critical Care: A Prospective Cohort Study." *Chest* 149 (5): 1146–54. https://doi.org/10.1016/j. chest.2015.12.015.

Laurant, Miranda, David Reeves, Rosella Hermens, Jose Braspenning, Richard Grol, and Bonnie Sibbald. 2004. "Substitution of Doctors by Nurses in Primary Care." Cochrane Database of Systematic Reviews 4 (CD001271). https://doi. org/10.1002/14651858.CD001271.pub2.

Lenz, Elizabeth R., Mary O'Neil Mundinger, Robert L. Kane, Sarah C. Hopkins, and Susan X. Lin. 2004. "Primary Care Outcomes in Patients Treated by Nurse Practitioners or Physicians: Two-Year Follow-Up." *Medical Care Research and Review* 61 (3): 332–51. https://doi.org/10.1177/1077558704266821.

Lipsky, Michael. 1980. *Street-Level Bureaucracy*. New York: Russell Sage Foundation.

Loveman, Mara. 2005. "The Modern State and the Primitive Accumulation of Symbolic Power." *American Journal of Sociology* 110 (6): 1651–83. https://doi.org/10.1086/428688.

Lyu, Jiyoung, and Jeffrey A. Burr. 2016. "Socioeconomic Status across the Life Course and Cognitive Function among Older Adults: An Examination of the Latency, Pathways, and Accumulation Hypotheses." *Journal of Aging and Health* 28 (1): 40–67. https://doi.org/10.1177/0898264315585504.

Marmot, Michael. 2004. *The Status Syndrome: How Social Standing Affects Our Health and Longevity*. London: Bloomsbury.

Martínez-González, Nahara Anani, Sima Djalali, Ryan Tandjung, Flore Huber-Geismann, Stefan Markun, Michel Wensing, and Thomas Rosemann. 2014. "Substitution of Physicians by Nurses in Primary Care: A Systematic Review and Meta-analysis." *BMC Health Services Research* 14 (1): 214–30. https://doi.org/10.1186/1472-6963-14-214.

Massey, Douglas S., and Nancy A. Denton. 1993. *American Apartheid: Segregation and the Making of the Underclass*. Cambridge, MA: Harvard University Press.

Mishler, Elliot G. 1985. *The Discourse of Medicine: Dialectics of Medical Interviews*. Norwood, NJ: Ablex.

Morgen, Sandra. 2001. "The Agency of Welfare Workers: Negotiating Devolution, Privatization, and the Meaning of Self-Sufficiency." *American Anthropologist* 103 (3): 747–61. https://doi.org/10.1525/aa.2001.103.3.747.

Mundinger, Mary O'Neil, Robert L. Kane, Elizabeth R. Lenz, Annette M. Totten, Wei-Yann Tsai, Paul D. Cleary, William T. Friedewald, Albert L. Siu, and Michael L. Shelanski. 2000. "Primary Care Outcomes in Patients Treated by Nurse Practitioners or Physicians: A Randomized Trial." *JAMA: The Journal of the American Medical Association* 283 (1): 59–68. https://doi.org/10.1001/jama.283.1.59.

Naylor, Mary D., and Ellen T. Kurtzman. 2010. "The Role of Nurse Practitioners in Reinventing Primary Care." *Health Affairs* 29 (5): 893–99. https://doi.org/10.1377/hlthaff.2010.0440.

Nelson, Sioban, and Suzanne Gordon. 2006. "Introduction." In *The Complexities of Care: Nursing Reconsidered*, edited by Sioban Nelson and Suzanne Gordon, 1–12. Ithaca, NY: Cornell University Press.

Newhouse, Robin P., Julie Stanik-Hutt, Kathleen M. White, Meg Johantgen, Eric B. Bass, George Zangaro, Renee F. Wilson, Lily Fountain, Donald M. Steinwachs, Lou Heindel, and Jonathan P. Weiner. 2011. "Advanced Practice Nurse Outcomes 1990–2008: A Systematic Review." *Nursing Economic$* 29 (5): 230–50.

Newman, Katherine S. 2003. *A Different Shade of Gray: Midlife and Beyond in the Inner City*. New York: New Press.

Nightingale, Florence. 1860. *Notes on Nursing: What It Is, and What It Is Not*. London: Harrison and Sons.

——. 1865. *Suggestions on a System of Nursing for Hospitals in India*. London: Eyre & Spottiswoode. https://wellcomecollection.org/works/d8wf7fvt.

Norris, Pauline. 2001. "How 'We' Are Different from 'Them': Occupational Boundary Maintenance in the Treatment of Musculo-skeletal Problems." *Sociology of Health & Illness* 23 (1): 24–43.

Oakley, Ann. 2018. *The Sociology of Housework*. Reissue. Chicago: Policy Press.

Ohman-Strickland, Pamela A., A. John Orzano, Shawna V. Hudson, Leif I. Solberg, Barbara DiCiccio-Bloom, Dena O'Malley, Alfred F. Tallia, Bijal A. Balasubramanian, and Benjamin F. Crabtree. 2008. "Quality of Diabetes Care in Family Medicine Practices: Influence of Nurse-Practitioners and Physician's Assistants." *Annals of Family Medicine* 6 (1): 14–22. https://doi.org/10.1370/afm.758.

Olshansky, S. Jay, and A. Brian Ault. 1986. "The Fourth Stage of the Epidemiologic Transition: The Age of Delayed Degenerative Diseases." *Milbank Quarterly* 64 (3): 355–91. https://doi.org/10.2307/3350025.

O'Malley, Ann S., Amelia M. Bond, and Robert A. Berenson. 2011. "Rising Hospital Employment of Physicians: Better Quality, Higher Costs?" Issue Brief No. 136. Washington, DC: Center for Studying Heath System Change. http://www.hschange.org/CONTENT/1230/indexbe25.html?PRINT=1.

Omran, Abdel R. 1971. "The Epidemiologic Transition: A Theory of the Epidemiology of Population Change." *Milbank Memorial Fund Quarterly* 49 (4): 509–38. https://doi.org/10.2307/3349375.

——. 1977. "Epidemiologic Transition in the United States: The Health Factor in Population Change." *Population Bulletin* 32 (2): 1–42.

Ostwald, Sharon K., and Okwuoma Chi Abanobi. 1986. "Nurse Practitioners in a Crowded Marketplace: 1965–1985." *Journal of Community Health Nursing* 3 (3): 145–56.

Padavic, Irene, and Barbara F. Reskin. 2002. *Women and Men at Work*. Thousand Oaks, CA: SAGE.

Permut, Steven R. 2016. "AMA Statement on VA Proposed Rule on Advance Practice Nurses." Accessed October 10, 2016. https://www.ama-assn.org/press-center/ama-statements/ama-statement-va-proposed-rule-advanced-practice-nurses.

Polletta, Francesca, and Zaibu Tufail. 2016. "Helping without Caring: Role Definition and the Gender-Stratified Effects of Emotional Labor in Debt Settlement Firms." *Work and Occupations* 43 (4): 401–33. https://doi.org/10.1177/0730888416656031.

Radwin, Laurel E. 1996. "'Knowing the Patient': A Review of Research on an Emerging Concept." *Journal of Advanced Nursing* 23 (6): 1142–46. https://doi.org/10.1046/j.1365-2648.1996.12910.x.

Ramsay, Janice A., John K. McKenzie, and David G. Fish. 1982. "Physicians and Nurse Practitioners: Do They Provide Equivalent Health Care?" *American Journal of Public Health* 72 (1): 55–57.

Reverby, Susan. 1987a. *Ordered to Care: The Dilemma of American Nursing, 1850–1945*. Cambridge: Cambridge University Press.

——. 1987b. "A Caring Dilemma: Womanhood and Nursing in Historical Perspective." *Nursing Research* 36 (1): 5–11.

Rice, Angie H. 2000. "Interdisciplinary Collaboration in Health Care: Education, Practice, and Research." *National Academies of Practice Forum: Issues in Interdisciplinary Care* 2 (1): 59–73.

Ridgeway, Cecilia L. 1997. "Interaction and the Conservation of Gender Inequality: Considering Employment." *American Sociological Review* 62 (2): 218–35. https://doi.org/10.2307/2657301.

Rosenberg, Charles E. 1995. *The Care of Strangers: The Rise of America's Hospital System*. Baltimore, MD: Johns Hopkins University Press.

Roth, Julius A., and Dorothy J. Douglas. 1983. *No Appointment Necessary: The Hospital Emergency Department in the Medical Services World*. New York: Irvington.

Salsberg, Edward, Leo Quigley, Nicholas Mehfoud, Kimberley Acquaviva, Karen Wyche, and Shari Sliwa. 2017. *Profile of the Social Work Workforce.* Washington, DC: George Washington University Health Workforce Institute.

Sandelowski, Margarete. 2000. *Devices and Desires: Gender, Technology, and American Nursing.* Raleigh, NC: University of North Carolina Press.

Schleef, Debra J. 2006. *Managing Elites: Professional Socialization in Law and Business Schools.* Lanham, MD: Rowman & Littlefield.

Schram, Sanford F., and Basha Silverman. 2012. "The End of Social Work: Neoliberalizing Social Policy Implementation." *Critical Policy Studies* 6 (2): 128–45. https://doi.org/10.1080/19460171.2012.689734.

Schwartz, Mark D. 2012. "Health Care Reform and the Primary Care Workforce Bottleneck." *Journal of General Internal Medicine* 27 (4): 469–72. https://doi.org/10.1007/s11606-011-1921-4.

Silver, Henry K., Loretta C. Ford, and Susan G. Steady. 1967. "A Program to Increase Health Care for Children: The Pediatric Nurse Practitioner Program." *Pediatrics* 39 (5): 756–60.

Smith, David Barton. 1990. "Population Ecology and the Racial Integration of Hospitals and Nursing Homes in the United States." *Milbank Quarterly* 68 (4): 561–96. https://doi.org/10.2307/3350194.

Smith, David Barton, Zhanlian Feng, Mary L. Fennell, Jacqueline S. Zinn, and Vincent Mor. 2007. "Separate and Unequal: Racial Segregation and Disparities in Quality across U.S. Nursing Homes." *Health Affairs* 26 (5): 1448–58. https://doi.org/10.1377/hlthaff.26.5.1448.

Smith, Steven Rathgeb, and Michael Lipsky. 2009. *Nonprofits for Hire: The Welfare State in the Age of Contracting.* Cambridge, MA: Harvard University Press.

Soss, Joe, Richard C. Fording, and Sanford F. Schram. 2011. *Disciplining the Poor: Neoliberal Paternalism and the Persistent Power of Race.* Chicago: University of Chicago Press.

Spector, Malcolm, and John I. Kitsuse. 2017. *Constructing Social Problems.* New York: Routledge.

Stacey, Clare L. 2005. "Finding Dignity in Dirty Work: The Constraints and Rewards of Low-Wage Home Care Labour." *Sociology of Health & Illness* 27 (6): 831–54. https://doi.org/10.1111/j.1467-9566.2005.00476.x.

——. 2011. *The Caring Self: The Work Experiences of Home Care Aides.* Ithaca, NY: Cornell University Press.

Stanek Kilbourne, Barbara, Paula England, George Farkas, Kurt Beron, and Dorothea Weir. 1994. "Returns to Skill, Compensating Differentials, and Gender Bias: Effects of Occupational Characteristics on the Wages of White Women and Men." *American Journal of Sociology* 100 (3): 689–719.

Stanik-Hutt, Julie, Robin P. Newhouse, Kathleen M. White, Meg Johantgen, Eric B. Bass, George Zangaro, Renee Wilson, Lily Fountain, Donald M. Steinwachs, Lou Heindel, and Jonathan P. Weiner. 2013. "The Quality and Effectiveness of Care Provided by Nurse Practitioners." *Journal for Nurse Practitioners* 9 (8): 492–500. e13. https://doi.org/10.1016/j.nurpra.2013.07.004.

Starr, Paul. 1984. *The Social Transformation of American Medicine: The Rise of a Sovereign Profession and the Making of a Vast Industry.* New York: Basic Books.

Stein, Leonard I. 1967. "The Doctor-Nurse Game." *Archives of General Psychiatry* 16 (6): 699–703.

Stein, Leonard I., David T. Watts, and Timothy Howell. 1990. "The Doctor-Nurse Game Revisited." *New England Journal of Medicine* 322 (8): 546–49.

Sudano, Joseph J., and David W. Baker. 2006. "Explaining US Racial/Ethnic Disparities in Health Declines and Mortality in Late Middle Age: The Roles of

Socioeconomic Status, Health Behaviors, and Health Insurance." *Social Science & Medicine* 62 (4): 909–22. https://doi.org/10.1016/j.socscimed.2005.06.041.

Sudnow, David. 1967. *Passing On: The Social Organization of Dying.* Englewood Cliffs, NJ: Prentice Hall.

Tanner, Christine A., Patricia Benner, Catherine Chesla, and Deborah R. Gordon. 1993. "The Phenomenology of Knowing the Patient." *Image: The Journal of Nursing Scholarship* 25 (4): 273–80. https://doi.org/10.1111/j.1547-5069.1993.tb00259.x.

Thomeer, Mieke Beth, Stipica Mudrazija, and Jacqueline L. Angel. 2015. "How Do Race and Hispanic Ethnicity Affect Nursing Home Admission? Evidence from the Health and Retirement Study." *Journals of Gerontology Series B: Psychological Sciences and Social Sciences* 70 (4): 628–38. https://doi.org/10.1093/geronb/gbu114.

Trotter, LaTonya. 2019. "'I'm Not a Doctor. I'm a Nurse': Reparative Boundary-Work in Nurse Practitioner Education." *Social Currents* 6 (2): 105–20. https://doi.org/10.1177/2329496518783683.

Villagrana, Marco A. 2018. "Medicare Graduate Medical Education Payments: An Overview." 10960. *In Focus.* Congressional Research Service. https://fas.org/sgp/crs/misc/IF10960.pdf.

Waitzkin, Howard. 1989. "A Critical Theory of Medical Discourse: Ideology, Social Control, and the Processing of Social Context in Medical Encounters." *Journal of Health and Social Behavior* 30 (2): 220–39. https://doi.org/10.2307/2137015.

Wald, Lillian D. 1902. "The Nurses' Settlement in New York." *American Journal of Nursing* 2 (8): 567–75. https://doi.org/10.2307/3401585.

———. 1915. *The House on Henry Street.* New York: Henry Holt.

Wallace, Steven. P., Lene Levy-Storms, Raynard S. Kington, and Ronald M. Andersen. 1998. "The Persistence of Race and Ethnicity in the Use of Long-Term Care." *Journals of Gerontology Series B: Psychological Sciences and Social Sciences* 53 (2): S104–112.

Welter, Barbara. 1966. "The Cult of True Womanhood: 1820–1860." *American Quarterly* 18 (2): 151–74. https://doi.org/10.2307/2711179.

West, Candace. 1984. *Routine Complications: Troubles with Talk between Doctors and Patients.* Bloomington: Indiana University Press.

Williams, David R. 2012. "Miles to Go before We Sleep: Racial Inequities in Health." *Journal of Health and Social Behavior* 53 (3): 279–95. https://doi.org/10.1177/0022146512455804.

Witz, Anne. 1990. "Patriarchy and Professions: The Gendered Politics of Occupational Closure." *Sociology* 24 (4): 675–90. https://doi.org/10.1177/0038038590024004007.

———. 1992. *Professions and Patriarchy.* New York: Routledge.

Wong, Carol A., Greta G. Cummings, and Lisa Ducharme. 2013. "The Relationship between Nursing Leadership and Patient Outcomes: A Systematic Review Update." *Journal of Nursing Management* 21 (5): 709–24. https://doi.org/10.1111/jonm.12116.

Yao, Li, and Stephanie A. Robert. 2008. "The Contributions of Race, Individual Socioeconomic Status, and Neighborhood Socioeconomic Context on the Self-Rated Health Trajectories and Mortality of Older Adults." *Research on Aging* 30 (2): 251–73. https://doi.org/10.1177/0164027507311155.

———. 2011. "Examining the Racial Crossover in Mortality between African American and White Older Adults: A Multilevel Survival Analysis of Race, Individual Socioeconomic Status, and Neighborhood Socioeconomic Context." *Journal of Aging Research* 2011 (article ID 132073). https://doi.org/10.4061/2011/132073.

Zerubavel, Eviatar. 1979. *Patterns of Time in Hospital Life.* Chicago: University of Chicago Press.

Index

(

Printed in the USA
CPSIA information can be obtained
at www.ICGtesting.com
CBHW020049010824
12532CB00006B/134